MEMOIRS OF

A former television producer and j
is a columnist and illustrator for British and Indian media. Her short fiction has been published in three continents, and is as full of mischief as her two young children.

MEMOIRS OF MY BODY

SHREYA SEN-HANDLEY

HarperCollins *Publishers* India

First published in India in 2017 by
HarperCollins *Publishers*

Copyright © Shreya Sen-Handley 2017
Illustration copyright © Shreya Sen-Handley 2017

P-ISBN: 978-93-5277-088-5
E-ISBN: 978-93-5277-089-2

2 4 6 8 10 9 7 5 3 1

Shreya Sen-Handley asserts the moral right to be identified
as the author of this work.

The views and opinions expressed in this book are the author's own and
the facts are as reported by her, and the publishers
are not in any way liable for the same.

All rights reserved. No part of this publication may be reproduced,
stored in a retrieval system, or transmitted, in any form or
by any means, electronic, mechanical, photocopying,
recording or otherwise, without the prior
permission of the publishers.

HarperCollins *Publishers*

A-75, Sector 57, Noida, Uttar Pradesh 201301, India
1 London Bridge Street, London, SE1 9GF, United Kingdom
2 Bloor Street East, Toronto, Ontario M4W 1A8, Canada
Lvl 13, 201 Elizabeth Street (PO Box A565, NSW, 1235),
Sydney NSW 2000, Australia
195 Broadway, New York, NY 10007, USA

Typeset in 11.5/14 Arno Pro at
SÜRYA, New Delhi

Printed and bound at
Thomson Press (India) Ltd

*This one's for my rock and two shiny pebbles,
with all my love*

Contents

Author's Note	ix
1. How Green Was My Valley	1
2. Popping the Cherry	17
3. Crimson Tide	32
4. May Day, May Day	46
5. Madness Becomes Her	57
6. You Taste of Chocolate, Girl	72
7. Hit Me Baby One More Time	86
8. Kiss a Few Frogs	103
9. Delhi's Underbelly	121
10. Bits and Bobs	136
11. Vee for Vagina (and Wanda, the Wilful Womb)	152
12. Nudity Begins at Home	166
13. Sex After Marriage aka SAM I AM	183
14. The Bouncy, Baleful World of Binky and Bonky	198
15. Death Rattles and Rolls On	217
16. Meltdowns for Mommies	234
Acknowledgements	253
References	255

Author's Note

Piglet looked around Hundred Acre Wood and thought, quite astutely, that it looked more like Sherwood Forest that fine summer morn. 'If fact and fiction are thrown together all higgledy-pig-gledy, what would you call it, Pooh?'

'I would call it fun, Piglet,' said Pooh wisely, sounding not a bit like a Bear of Very Little Brain. 'Some may call it auto-fiction.'

Piglet rolled this new term around in his head, trying to see if it worked for the thing he'd written. Deciding he liked it very much indeed, he yanked the lid off their celebratory jar of honey, pushing it towards his friend for his bear's share. Pooh dived in delightedly, even before he heard Piglet squeak 'enjoy'.

But the wind had carried Piglet's benediction to every other creature in the magically melding forest, and the fun was just about to begin.

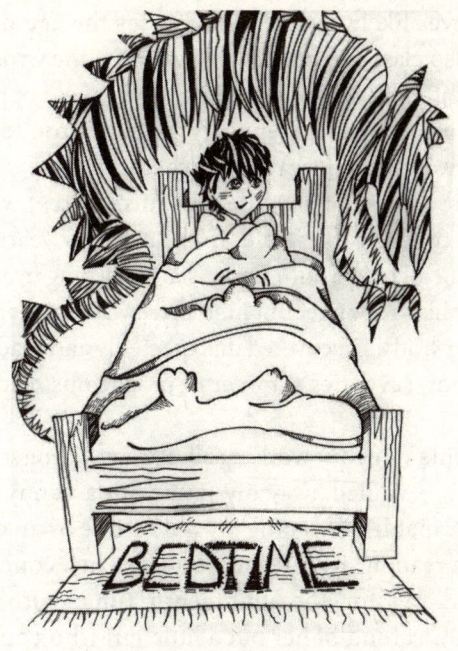

1

How Green Was My Valley

In the hierarchy of summers of discovery, the first scorcher came early.

I had joined 'proper' school that year and was in the middle of my first meanderingly long summer break, when I spotted the man who would usher in my coming of age. He walked into my world on a pair of weathered chappals and awakened the woman in me. Yes, in primary school. Don't jump the gun. Or reach for it. He didn't touch me. At least, not physically.

I called him 'Green Boy' because I didn't know his name

and was never likely to find out. Besides the age difference, there was also class between us. He was from the wrong side of the tracks. Literally. Beyond the little playing field opposite our home in Kolkata were perennially haze-enshrouded railway tracks that wound their way to nowhere.

Nowhere I knew, at any rate. Just turned six, I was on the brink of discovering the world. In the next few years, I would have traipsed all over South East Asia, absorbing everything it had to offer like a sponge. But first, there was another world to discover: my body. Discovered unexpectedly and inadvertently that long, hot, seventies summer of precocious reading. And Green Boy.

My parents were out working all day, my younger sister yet to arrive. So, I whiled away my time with a nanny who was kind but incapable of keeping my quick little brain occupied.

'Are you reading again?' she would ask me, concerned.

'Yes,' I'd say for the umpteenth time, with growing irritation. I was fond of her but a little girl who could not be fobbed off with her practised bribes of 'keeleeps', 'bishkoot' or sneaky half-hours of terrible television at the neighbour's house (because Baba had refused to buy us a set), was beyond her capabilities. 'Where are the pictures?' she would then ask suspiciously. She wasn't wrong to suspect something was afoot. It was a serious case of literary effrontery. I had outgrown picture books years ago, and on that dust-mote dappled afternoon, I was reading *To Kill a Mockingbird*.

And that was the least of it. That summer, I started reading books placed on shelves slightly above my head in the many bookcases in our house. These were the shelves for 'older kids'. As the oldest child in the house (and the only one), I decided that meant me. As I ingested rows of previously inaccessible books, some lines stuck, and I would repeat them to myself with delight. 'I'd rather take coffee than compliments just now,' I would say à la Jo March, while tottering through the hall in my mom's high heels.

The radio was the other constant in my life, but neither Rabindra Sangeet nor filmi tunes did anything for me. Jim Morrison though, heard just once and in passing, left me with a feeling I couldn't fathom. My ayah, on the other hand, listened to Bollywoodsy warbling from the minute my mother left to teach in the morning to the moment she heard that first footfall outside our door in the late afternoon. Those first footsteps shattering the quiet of the afternoon could have belonged to anyone, including the cleaner who dropped in to shift the dust around twice a day. In the middle of the day, after she had served me a lunch of rice and fish, the ayah would retire to her small room for an hour's kip, confident in the knowledge that I would happily spend the afternoon doing something quiet. Clearly, she was unaware that being quiet was often the worst thing an inquisitive child could be.

'If I were to sleep,' she would say as if she had any choice in the matter, 'what would you do?' At first, I would answer her truthfully. 'I will play with my one-and-a-half dolls.' (Baba didn't believe in buying those either) Then I moved on to the books, and mentioning them led to too many questions, even attempts at staying awake on her part. But when I discovered the delights of self-exploration, my answer went back to, 'I shall play.' She would nod off, reassured. And I did play, didn't I?

But for that to happen, Green Boy had to saunter into my life.

Some muggy afternoons, after finishing with the books within reach and the measly music on offer, I had little else to do but swing on the railings of our first-floor balcony, watching the cricket on the little patch of green ahead. Boys from the neighbourhood ran, dived and shouted with glee as I observed them quietly.

'Oi you monkey, the ball is racing to the boundary!'

'How do you expect me to see past your brother? He's bigger than your house!'

Then it would be fisticuffs before dusk, till the sweets shop owner walked over purposefully to clout one of the boys on the ear, which was the agreed signal for close of play.

I would watch all this, occasionally chortling to myself, turning my attention back to a book I was rereading (there was time to read and reread while Babloo, their slowest batsman, was at the crease) or cocking my head to hear the faint strains of music from the radio inside the house. If it was still on the same station, my ayah was asleep. One such afternoon, my eyes alighted on Green Boy and I grew up in nanoseconds.

He was a cricket-playing, little-else-doing young man. At six, even an imaginative six, I could not think of a fancier name than that. But then there was nothing fancy about Green Boy, and the sobriquet fitted him to a T. And it was a tee, his green, long-suffering tee that I named him after. You see, he never wore anything else. It was this, and a pair of khaki flares to go with it. As it was the late seventies, he had bristling sideburns to match. Maybe not green, but still flared and flora-like, taking over his narrow young face. He was in his teens: a distant god.

I watched him from my balcony as he played badly, oblivious to my scrutiny. Our paths only ever crossed at the sweets shop, which I was sent to regularly to stock up on my family's rosogolla (and related) requirements. Little did they know what danger they were exposing me to. No, not from the fellow himself but from the vistas opening up in my mind. Had they known the overcooked, overblown saga of love and rebellion that my head and heart were spawning, they would have thought twice about sending me to 'Lapu'r Lyangchas' so often.

Occasional conversations between me and Green Boy went like this:

'Dada-Boudi ki kinte pathieyecche?'

'Rosogolla.'

'Baah. Rosogollar moton mishti aar hoyena.'

And I would blush a deep red and scurry home with a 'bhnar' of rosogolla, convinced he'd indirectly admitted to a soft spot for my sweet nature. He soon entered my dreams by day and by night. The former were innocuous enough to start with. It was in the latter that he started doing strange things to me I couldn't name. I would toss and turn through the night and find wet streaks in my underpants in the morning. I worried initially that I had gone back to bed-wetting, but then I had a waking dream about him. A daydream, where he did indescribable, but not unlikeable, things to me. And suddenly, I had a whole new set of worries. Including those wet streaks which were now revealed to be not-wee. But also, wonderfully, secret delights to indulge in.

Butterflies in My Tummy

One drowsy afternoon, as I read *Daddy-Long-Legs* in my secluded corner, I was visited by my nocturnal hauntings. I held my breath as it filled my head, then travelled downwards. Green Boy sits with me under the lonely tree on the cricket field. There is no one else (I am infatuated, not an exhibitionist). He touches me. Then he touches me *there*. Yes, there. That place that never struck me as a 'there' till this moment, when the strangest sensations are triggered by his touch. But not his touch; they are my own. As it had been night after night without my really knowing.

My fingers didn't do much at first. They just brushed. Then felt. Then brushed again. Finally, fingers inside my little girl pants, which then skittered away as if singed. But delved back in again. How could you not when it made you feel like you didn't know you could?

And it spread with each stroke. It invaded my tummy. Like butterflies with their wingtips on fire, grazing my insides and setting them alight. Under cover of the dark, and a light sheet that you could just about bear having draped over you in the summer months, I found that positioning my 'pash baalish' between my thighs felt rather good. If I moved gently against it, it felt even better. And if I thought of Green Boy while doing that, those flaming butterflies didn't just flutter, they dive-bombed into my gut like blazing balls of fire.

Suddenly, inanimate objects which could be balled and slid between my legs took on a new life, pushed into a service they hadn't known before. I didn't know they were pretend-penises of course. What, after all, was a penis? There were no boys in my home. Nor did I ever introduce anything inside myself. A natural squeamishness stepped in to prevent that. That this was an activity which seemed to scandalize people the world over, I had no idea at all. I quite innocently relished the sensations I'd begun to discover. And then, I couldn't wait till bedtime anymore. I found nooks and crannies around the house to which I could melt away.

A particular favourite in the somnolent afternoons, when the world stood still, was the space behind the naked bed frame, left leaning on its side against the bright yellow wall of the spare bedroom. I scavenged around the house to make my den comfortable (and not just for *that*; it was perfect for reading too, especially books that worried my nanny). A purloined 'madur' and my trusty 'paash baalish' made it a comfortable hideaway for all sorts of activities.

Till I got caught and my pleasurable little world shattered into tiny shards of shame.

Growing Up Guilty

My comeuppance came swiftly, and it was harsh. I was discovered en flagrante delicto with my paash baalish and told in no uncertain terms how unnatural and disgusting it was.

'Who does that at this age? This, this, MONKEY business!' my horrified mother scowled forbiddingly at me. At that moment, I just wanted to disappear. Forever. I wanted to dissolve into a dark corner (but not the one I'd just been found in) and never emerge. Suddenly, the splendid feeling I had learnt to give myself became this dirty thing that defined me. It clung to me like a bad smell. Monkey, monkey, monkey, went the voice in my head. And continued for a good twenty years after.

So, I'm not going on Oprah or anything, people (only because she hasn't asked), but why does this happen? Why is this burden of shame, where nothing shameful has been done, laid on each of us? For years, the whole business of sex, especially my own sexual urges, would be tainted by this view that it was filthy, bestial, and one of my many failings. I would grow up hating my body and worrying about sex. My anxieties ranged from whether it was right to want sex to wondering if anyone would want me at all. I saw myself as a deviant, with a head crammed with unduly sexual thoughts and a body that found those thoughts so pleasurable. I didn't know I was far from alone because in India, no one discussed such things. The Birds and Bees talk, if it was given, was cursory and explained nothing.

Mumble, mumble, mumble. Much throat clearing and minute finger scrutiny. 'So, you get that don't you, son? Anu, dinner! We are done here.' Head rub and exit. Child stares after his father, aghast. That's all the dude knows? I know more than him!

If the BB talk skimmed over sex, it certainly never touched upon masturbation. That only came up when a parent angrily stumbled upon the fact that their perfect little girl or boy had discovered its joys. 'Badmaash bachha!' they splutter at the cowering child, desperately trying to hide her offending hands behind her back. 'What are you doing to *our* good name behaving like that? What gives you these ideas? These looj western ideas? No more Enid Blyton for you!'

At that moment, they screw him or her up forever. This was the point at which they should have said, 'I know what you're going through. I've been there too. Because no one told me the things I'm about to tell you; I went through half my life unsure about sexual pleasures, especially the ones I give myself. But I don't want you to go through that. I want you to know now what you're doing is not just normal, everybody does it. And it certainly doesn't make you a bad person.'

But they don't, do they? And heck, what chance have they got of getting it right when the Mother of all Fathers, God, didn't? If He'd cast an indulgent eye over the snake and apple and a furiously blushing Adam, and decided to be cool about it, it would have been a different story for the billions who followed after. But noooo, he had to go all funny and thunderbolty and get-out-of-paradise-y about it. Playing with your snake or your apple became a sin forever more. And now it's the norm for parents to frown upon it even when doctors and more importantly, Hollywood, tell them otherwise.

'I did a fair bit of masturbating when I was young,' said father to son in *American Pie*. 'I used to call it stroking the salami, yeah, you know, pounding the old pud.'

Which is pretty much what Freud said in 'Three Essays On the Theory of Sexuality' (1905): 'One feature of the popular view of the sexual instinct is that it is absent in childhood and only awakens in the period of life described as puberty. This, however, is not merely a simple error but one that has had grave consequences.'

Indeed. But did anyone listen?

Those Kinds of Girls

A friend liked to play turtle. She couldn't have been more than six either. She liked to curl up over a cushion, and then ducking her head and arching her back, she'd do this weird humping thing like a dog. Just like that, any old time of the day, completely innocently. It could be in the middle of a game of tag or something, and the rest of us who'd gathered to play at her house would carry on with our game, leaving her to it. We weren't even curious. Many years later, I realized she had been masturbating. And it struck me only because a conversation from long ago floated back across the ether.

'Why are your palms so red, Reema?' I asked her one day, rather worried about her. Just turned six, I was at the age when empathy blossoms in children.

'Mamoni hit them,' she said unhappily.

'Why?' I asked, scared because I knew I was guilty of all sorts of things from sneaking sweets to that new thing I enjoyed. That new thing that I *sensed* would be disapproved of if it were discovered.

'I was being a turtle,' she said, with downturned face and blazing ear-tips. I knew immediately what she meant. I recognized that it was a lot like my own trysts with the paash baalish. I wondered why she was struck for it but then forgot all about it till my own moment of reckoning.

We were told we were freaks and we believed it. We certainly never compared notes on it, not in the India I grew up in. A chance encounter in a London bar with an old school friend finally started us off on the subject of youthful indiscretions. Liberated women as we had by then become, we began laughing about male and then female wanking. We talked of girls who had let it slip that they'd slipped things in when the urge overtook them, like us, at a relatively young age. And the disproportionately harsh chastisement that inevitably followed. 'They found me with my hand up my pants,' she cackled about her own experience. Then sobering, she said, 'I wasn't laughing then. I got the dressing down of a lifetime. Everything was thrown at me, from how unnatural it was to … how natural, in a strange way. That animals did it, so, I shouldn't.'

As a result of the condemnation, we grow into adults seriously screwed up about sex. In India, the 'don't talk about it, don't do it in a consensual, open, grown-up way' approach to sex has ruined it for far too many, for-effing-ever. Sex is 'bad', so it has to be done surreptitiously. It's wicked, so it has to be pushed upon unwilling partners as punishment. And instead of happy, openly loving couples, we wind up with rapidly multiplying cases of rape and molestation. The National Crime Records Bureau found that in 2014, ninety-three women were raped every day, up significantly from the previous year, despite all the promises made after the infamous Delhi rape of 2012. Yay.

What's bizarre though is that in the sexually liberated west, masturbation is not talked about much either. Parents continue to skim over it as best as they can. Little boys may get a token talk but little girls get nada. And although popular Western culture is hardly puritanical, female masturbation is a no-go zone. As if it doesn't happen or is only practised by the depraved. Popular sitcoms *Family Guy* or *The Inbetweeners* are famous for their obsession with male masturbation, but stop a minute to think about the mainstream female equivalent and what do you get? Nup.

Men masturbating is all in a day's work, and a staple of many a crass, mainstream comedy. A woman masturbating, however, is sinister, unnatural and unhealthy. Why else don't we see it on everyday TV or in films? You're thinking about it, aren't you? You're thinking *hard*. It's … erm … rather obvious. What's not obvious is why masturbating women are considered such a threat to humanity. Two consecutive sex scenes were shot for *Reign*, the American teen television show on Mary, Queen of Scots. The first involved a girl masturbating, and the second, her coercion into sex by an older, powerful man who discovers her touching herself. But only one got the chop – no prizes for guessing which one.

Masturbation, especially of the feminine kind, is clearly a greater evil than rape or paedophilia. TV critic Rachel Grate fumed, 'It's time we as a society discuss why we're concerned a masturbation scene in a show for teens would create awkward conversations for parents, while a rape scene would apparently need no explanation at all.' Why is it such a taboo topic still? Tracy Clark-Flory on the news site *Salon* explains it as society being 'thoroughly comfortable with women's bodies being sexualized – but not so much with women being sexual.'[1]

In other words, men want us for sex but won't have us want sex for ourselves. Besides, sexual pleasure without a man isn't even possible.

Or is it?

Mad-sturbation

We've established that a wanker (I mean a masturbating man) is funny at worst. A woman doing 'it' is dirty, demonic or hysterical. Hysteria itself, derived from the word 'hyster' or uterus in Greek, was regarded by the Ancients as an exclusively feminine mental disorder that sprang from a 'sex-starved womb'. Go forward many hundreds of years to the Victorian Age and they were no wiser (by choice, don't you know). Sexual emancipation in women was seen as madness, and masturbation one of its symptoms. Isaac Baker-Brown, erstwhile president of the Medical Society of London proposed, persuasively at the time, clitoridectomies as the remedy. Joseph Howe agreed, claiming masturbation mangled women's bits, 'I have seen cases where the labia resembled the ear of a small spaniel.' He was convinced masturbating women were not only prone to hysteria but nymphomania as well. The only cure for this 'uncontrollable appetite for lascivious pleasures, exhibited in public and private, without regard to time, place, or surroundings was marriage, or the amputation of the clitoris.'[2] Since such women already had their legs spread at all times, they were practically begging the good doctor to reach in and ... snip.

Another school of quackery decided the answer lay in feeding the need of the questing fanny with artificially induced orgasms. Joseph Granville invented the first vibrator, a clunky contraption that these men used to control and even damage women with scary, wanton wombs[3]. But boy, did they end up with egg on their faces! Today, smoother, softer, gentler versions give women *so* much pleasure. From the oh-my-how-large-is-that (but I'll try it on for size) dildos to tiny vibrators-in-underwear for women-on-the-go, sex toys come in all shapes, sizes, textures, temperatures and flavours.

Use it any time of the day, anywhere at all. And without any involvement from a man (oh except the George Clooneys and Orlando Blooms blossoming in your head). So, in an appropriately Mary Shelley-esque turn of events, the monster is now our slave and its creator out in the cold, unless we let him in. Orgasmic justice, eh?

And now we're talkin'. Amidst a right-wing backlash to her candid account of youthful experimentation in her book *Not That Kind of Girl*, Lena Dunham took to Twitter to slug it out, 'If you were a little kid and never looked at another little kid's vagina, well, congrats to you. I told a story about being a weird seven-year-old. I bet you have some too, Old Men, that I'd rather not hear.'[4] A popular social media movement followed, overflowing with masturbating women who would not be muzzled anymore. An Arab Spring of the vagina. They called it Those Kinds of Girls. Because we all are. Even men.

Birds Do It, Bees Do It

Maybe not, but I have it on good authority that primates, our nearest cousins, most certainly do. Perhaps Ma was just being scientifically correct when she called it 'monkey business' rather than trying to shame me. But, in fact, it's not restricted to monkeys or even mammals. Pretty much everything that walks (flies/swims) the earth does it. They fondle their bits, use implements, even do each other. Professor David Linden gleefully recorded 'the most creative form of animal masturbation' as that of the male bottlenose dolphin, which 'wrapped live, wriggling eels around its penis'[5].

When we wank, we are furtive, guilt-ridden and terrified of discovery. But not animals, who are so at ease with it, they could have been born to do it. Because they are, and so are WE. Like the good doctor Freud said, 'The new-born child brings with it the germs of sexual feelings'[6]. And that doesn't make monkeys out of us. It just makes us human. But even as men like Darwin took us forward several millennia in our understanding of living creatures, many other Victorians were busy putting the clock back. And because many modern Indians cling to a Victorian world-view, I am allowed a rant about this peculiar period in history.

Hide the Piano Legs

What can you expect from an era that found uncovered piano legs provocative? Women were stuffed into straitjackets and homosexuals into closets. Children were seen (but only at teatime, on a leash) and never heard. Stern warnings were issued about the terrible consequences – from paralysis to heart disease to madness – of the 'life-wrecking sin' of masturbation.

These were accompanied by harsh restraints and punishments devised to discourage children. Sex-perv, oops, I meant sex-pert William Robinson endorsed thrashing the desire out of children, as beatings were the only language their basic intelligence could process, according to him. 'Never spank the masturbating child though,' he warned, 'they may enjoy it.' He also advocated tying kids to their beds and clamping 'specially made metal appliances on their genitals' to stop them touching themselves. Nor was he alone in encouraging this monstrous mistreatment of perfectly normal, utterly innocent children. Dr Kellog (cereal offender, you might say) recommended mutilating with 'red hot wires' children who were caught masturbating.

But even more terrifying than the punishments themselves is the idea that some of those punishments sounded like sexual abuse. The alarming conclusion almost everyone looking into these practices has arrived at is that 'correcting' masturbation in children may have been a convenient cover for paedophilia. If rapid downturns in health, alongside the sudden surfacing of psychological and behavioural problems in children were touted as symptoms of masturbation, they were also scream-out-loud signs of sex abuse.[7] This abuse was neither detected nor stopped, while people busied themselves punishing already traumatized children.

Did all this end with the Victorians though, considering how misinformed and morbidly afraid of masturbation we still are? How many of these quacks are still around, operating in hole-in-the-wall establishments in the small towns and villages of India? How many of us, although shocked by the punishment detailed above, still chide our children for masturbating or, at the very least, squirm when it's mentioned? Well, I had to deal with it recently. And I squirmed too but then I decided to do it differently.

'Mommy,' my six-year-old son asked, 'why does my tiddler grow fat sometimes?'

'Because you're growing up, and so is your body.'

'It buzzes as well.'

'Buzzes?'

'Does it, erm, buzz when you spot certain things ... like pretty girls?'

'No, Mommy, dinosaurs,' he said happily, 'it buzzes when I see dinosaurs.'

I stifled a laugh, telling him that it was fine but things could change with time, and to never worry or be embarrassed by things like that. I also told him to be comfortable with his body and enjoy everything about it. When he went to bed under his dinosaur duvet that night, I could see he was at peace with his tiddler's propensity for getting fat as well as buzzing. And though I knew he might be reaching for it the moment he heard my footsteps fading, I was happy too, happy that in being supportive, I had broken away from the millions of parents who get it wrong.

But breaking away comes at a price.

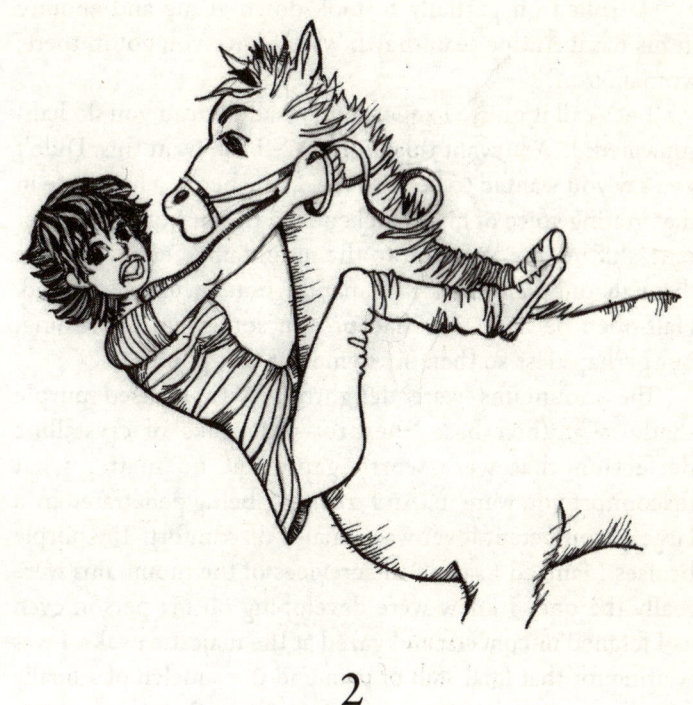

2

Popping the Cherry

'Gerroff!'

I'd been muttering for a while, not at all happy with how that promised earthshaking first experience was shaping up for me. Nothing shook except my resolve to stay the course. I needed a breather. So, I used what remained of my nearly crushed lungs to bellow. I also shoved at his vast body heaving atop me in the hope that he might shift some of his weight for even just a second, allowing me to breathe.

He rolled off partially to look down at me and enquire in his nasal Antipodean drawl, 'What have you got in there, woman, iron?'

'Let's call it quits,' I squeaked (what else can you do half-squashed?). 'You want this, right? We both want this. Didn't you say you wanted to be with me ...' he began a harangue in that grating voice of his. I chickened in the face of yet another rant, shifting my attention to the mountains I could glimpse through our half-open Kathmandu hotel window instead. Half-open because they had proven somewhat unyielding, but perhaps less so than my hymen at that point.

The mountains were delightful. With bruised purple shadows at their base, they rose to peaks of crystalline perfection that were worth gaping at no matter what discomfort you were in. And trust me, being penetrated by a large, incompetent lover was a major discomfort. The purple bruises I fancied I saw in the crevices of the mountains were really the ones I knew were developing on my person even as I feigned unconcern and gazed at the majestic peaks. I was waiting for that final stab of pain and the squelch of a finally torn hymen to tell me my ordeal was over. Because ordeal is what it had become.

I rummaged around in the recesses of my mind trying to remember how I had got there. What made me think this large, quivering, puce-coloured individual was *the* one? And *that* voice, grunting in my ear – HOW had I found that attractive? 'Jesus, woman' he was fulminating again, '*You* ain't my first but I sure as hell never encountered a plug-piece as stubborn as yours.' No, I ain't your first and wish you weren't mine, I thought to myself. His drawl started a slow burn of annoyance somewhere in my tummy, as did his round, red face hovering over mine, sweaty from the Herculean task he was labouring over: robbing me of my cherry.

So this was it? *This* had spawned a million love songs and romance novels? This clunky coming together was meant to make bells ring and angels sing in time with the awkward mashing of pelvic equipment? I could hear no angels or birds. From the street below our window rose the sounds of tooting auto-rickshaws and the pitter-patter of tourist feet, off to a pagoda or casino, the oblivion of their choice. And inside our room, there was no celestial music either. All that could be heard above my rising inner voice was the gritting of teeth (mine) and the revolting slap of flab (his) against firm flesh (mine). Not what I had signed up for at all!

Looking into the faux French mirror across the room I had been resolutely avoiding, my stomach lurched. I had been averting my gaze with good reason. At twenty-three, I didn't have to worry about what I'd see of my body in the looking glass. My tiny frame was taut and mocha-brown. I wouldn't make it to any centrefolds but there was nothing to embarrass me either. The problem was that *I couldn't look myself in the eye*.

Nor did I dare look at him. I worried that if I caught sight of his body wobbling in the mirror, it would weaken my resolve to go through with this. But then a treacherous little voice whispered in my head, isn't that what you really, really want? You don't want to do this, you don't want to be here at all! I squirmed unhappily. Though not much squirming was possible, pinned down as I was. This was love, I told myself sternly, and while right now wasn't pretty, we'd had our moments. With that, I resubmitted myself to his bucking and heaving and getting nowhere.

It was the fear of getting nowhere that had brought me to this room in Kathmandu, at the roof of the world, that lurid evening. Puce man, mocha woman, purple mountains and chintzy pink hotel room. Pretty colours that didn't work in the mix. Where does it come from, not the colours, but this overwhelming fear women start entertaining at the age of twenty-something, that life is passing them by? From that reliable source of good advice and intentions: society (aka Narrow-minded Tattlers and Nosey Parkers 'R' Us), of course! The clock is ticking, we're told. Get on with it, we're urged. If you haven't snagged a man and bred a brood before you're thirty, you're a failure, they warn. And while the age at which you hit haghood may have changed, the pressure to marry and breed has not. You may be allowed a few more years before the shrill cries to couple dog your every step, but dog them they will. Ain't it a bitch.

But because they start later, they feel a greater sense of urgency in hammering the message home, so you still get the same blackmail-derision-anxiety onslaught but in a stronger, concentrated form. Like gin, they slowly reduce the sweeter tonicky element as you get older. But gin is good for you (made of berries, right?), which nagging born of a parochial worldview could never be. Truth is, the nagging was never about getting women on the baby train at the right time. It's about ensuring society controls women's sexuality (knock 'em up early and they won't sleep around), careers (knock 'em up early and they'll never wrest power) and peace of mind (keep 'em panicky and they'll never focus on no.1). The world wants you tied up in knots, matrimonial and otherwise, before you can do any damage to the established order of things. So, you have to saddle yourself with a man, any man, regardless of whether he's right for you. A man is a man is a whole man by himself. A woman is a pathetic part-person without her 'better half'.

At twenty-three, I was doing exceptionally well at my chosen career of broadcast journalism, having achieved regional head status when many others my age were still fetching their seniors' chai. But I was forever being reminded that I didn't have a man in my life. 'Tomar toh keu neyi, na?' asked a friend's mom, dewy-eyed with concern. 'Um' I said, 'I have family and friends. Did you mean ...' 'A man! I meant a man. You haven't found one like Sona has.' But, but Sona answers the phone in a dingy front office and has nothing else to do, I was tempted to say. Still, Sona was a friend, though for how much longer I couldn't say. But the Mother of all Nags (and Sona) wasn't finished. 'Ma ke bolo chhele khuje dite. From a good phamily and phaine shkool. Engineer hote hobe, topper hote hobe ...'

I knew that list by heart anyway. With minor variations, it was the same for every Indian woman 'of marriageable age', which is anything less than thirty. The *man* doesn't have to be young, of course. He doesn't have to be kind or responsible. Or even bright. It doesn't matter if he's lost his hair or teeth and acquired a pot belly. All he has to do is bring home the paneer. Paneer and not juicy, meaty, delightful bacon. And not even all of it, because the wife's gotta pull her weight too (and then some). Why is his earning potential all that matters when he's unlikely to be the sole breadwinner? It may have been the most important quality at one time but not anymore.

And the woman, though often reluctant to reconcile herself to as little as society would like, really doesn't expect the earth from her man. Women, you see, have something called sense. Of course, they want their men to possess qualities they consider important! Some of my friends desired kindness most of all. I was not so mature; I wanted a connection. I needed a guy who'd 'get' me. Not too much to ask for, surely? But men. Sigh. Men want their women to be a long, long list of unlikely things that few mortal women are. And never all at once. Men are *encouraged* to make these outrageous demands. Because in India, if the woman falls short, her parents may be persuaded to cough up some dowry.

The usual demands then, in order of importance:

1. Light skin: We take light and dark very literally, the Vedic sages that we are. And which good woman has ever had dark skin? Oh, only several million Indian women, but never mind, we will still demand the impossible and drive our women to chemically alter their skin.
2. Long, straight hair: Hair should look like a jet waterfall. Just like Indian women have generally dusky skin, they also tend to have wavy hair – billows of beautiful, dark hair that's rarely dead straight. Also, it must be kept long. It's a vile rebellion to shear it off. Unfeminine. Un-Indian. You could just as well be throwing your vagina away. So I have. Not the vagina.
3. Tall: The lady's gotta be tall, though the average Indian man is 5'4. No matter. We will keep asking for unattainable things so we grind her self-esteem into the ground and maybe snag a dowry from her grateful parents, relieved we are taking their undesirable daughter off their hands.
4. Beauty: All of the above are absolutely essential to beauty, naturally. Who ever heard of a small, short-haired, dark-skinned *beauty*? Now that's an oxymoron. And a laugh. We are not content with the above though. We want a face of pearly symmetry. The slightest quirk might confer character on it, see, and we'll have no truck with character. Also, not a single one of our beauties have that symmetry we

keep pretending they have, not even Aishwarya with rounded face and the slight hook to her nose, but we will turn our noses up at our long-nosed, short-chinned, limpid-eyed beauties all the same or if they are fair-skinned, we will claim their faces harbour no imperfections. Confused? We are not. We never are. We are Indian and can't be wrong.

5. Domestication: Like dogs, this is essential in women. Women who don't cook, sew or clean up after you are hardly women and cannot be considered for marriage (phew, right?).

6. Uncomplaining, accommodating, obedient: No man should be questioned in his own home. Least of all by the Little Woman (little in terms of her mind. We know she has to be tall). She should hang on to his every word, follow every instruction and what's the occasional slight or insult as long as she's allowed to grace his home? Or his parents' home, as the case often is.

7. Exam topper, big earner: She should be all of that too. It's absolutely necessary she study science at university but not that she have a rational bent of mind (god forbid). In fact, she should pay close attention to what God forbids and pray to him twice a day. That is, when she's not throwing herself at her godlike husband's feet. Actual intelligence is not important because (and in this I agree), she'd only show him up. And she doesn't need it anyway to earn the big money that will keep her husband and his family in style.

8. Tagore-ability: This applies only to the Bengali community but is an absolute must for them. If you don't spout Tagore, or rant ad infinitum on how he's

best in the world at everything, just everything, then you don't have a hope in hell of snagging your own Kobi Guru. Because that's who your Bong bloke thinks he is, though he can't write, is tone deaf, and hasn't an ounce of T's vision. He has a scraggly beard and that's enough. And you? You better make sure you like wearing saris with red borders, flowers in your hair and out-simpering your man.

This list is *much* longer. Just eight asks on a man's list? How could you even think that was all? No, this is just a taster and that's all I needed, because I've failed miserably. Fulfilling not even one of the above criteria (Oh, OK, I was a big earner for a while). So, no IIM/IIT-topping Ganesh-lookalike for me.

I may be allowed to dredge for the dregs, of course (but are they the dregs? Are they? Or does Indian society have a cockeyed way of valuing people; women as well as men?). But if I refused to settle for the little I was told I could expect, who should I hold out for? Who, after all, is Mr Right? Is he that dashing, handsome and chivalrous dude from books and songs and films? Even Mr Darcy was flawed. So, if I was ready to find someone, I was ready to compromise a wee bit too. My body told me to. And when it wasn't, the meddling mausis did. But there are compromises and then there are compromises. I still wanted something outside the box. Whoever heard me obviously thought I meant too big for a box. So I got Duncan.

He was Kiwi. Flightless, as it turned out, like the bird. Too big and too unimaginative. And yet, he had seemed just the opposite at the beginning. The soul of sensitivity when we first started corresponding, he seemed to understand my rebellious, searching nature. He wrote me poems. Just for me, he said. He told me the sad story of his cerebral aneurism and uncaring ex-girlfriend who left him when the former was discovered, and I duly fell for it.

I cried over his tragedy. I was sent *old* pictures of a trim, young man playing cricket for a county side in New Zealand. He was doing a PhD on World War Two nurses, he said (turned out it was nurses in general he was studying, and not for a PhD). He would be spending a few months working in Kolkata. I was excited. I made arrangements. Over the months of talking, we'd grown close. More than close, words of love had been spoken. He had a way with words and an accent that stirred me. Right up to the day it began to annoy me. In the blurred photos sent, I discerned long-lashed blue eyes. And jowls. But that was a small matter of exercise. He clearly hadn't had time after his aneurism op. He had had to give up cricket too. In fact, he was taking a break from his dissertation. Just when I'd begun to wonder which bit of what he'd originally told me still applied, he arrived in Kolkata.

At the airport, I watched aghast as he trundled towards me. He had warned me he was out-of-shape, but I didn't know he meant out-of-human-into-zeppelin shape. He had a shock of orange hair. And long-lashed blue eyes. That at least was real, I thought. Or was it, I panicked. Maybe it's mascara, maybe it's Maybelline. But then I remembered the wonderful connection we shared. And the many heart-warming, insightful, exciting conversations we'd had over the last few months, and I melted a little. No, a lot. Despite his looks. Who was I to judge someone on looks?

'Hello,' I said stepping up to him. And he grabbed me in a big bear hug. I could smell the deodorant on him, a nice change from Indian men at the time. Then he said he wasn't feeling well, that he felt an aneurism coming on, and so, despite the hotel room I had booked for him, he came home with me.

Over the weeks of getting to know him in Kolkata (but not TOO well, we are talking Kolkata after all, where even the walls have eyes and ears. and a very big mouth), I decided that a serious relationship may be possible despite my initial disappointment. We fixed on a teeny-weeny Kathmandu to Kanyakumari (or thereabouts) crawl to cement our relationship, heading south for the marvels of Mahabalipuram and the peace of Pondicherry, and finishing with the coconut-chutney-laden culinary delights, colonial ruins and bustling temples of colourful, cacophonous Chennai.

On the road though, without the buffer of family and friends and the constant proximity it allowed us, I was no longer sure about going further with him. Kathmandu I'd do, but him? I was finding out who he really was and didn't like it. While wandering through the glorious ruins of ancient Mahabalipuram, kicking up sand and quaffing a kulfi, he stopped me in my happy tracks by suddenly and peevishly complaining that flesh and blood Indian women were not as stacked as their stone counterparts (he should see me now in my well-padded forties).

In Chennai, every time we sat down to eat what looked like the most mouth-watering meal in some spectacular location, by the sea or overlooking a humming, vividly painted temple, I'd stop to admire the sights, only to find the food gone when I turned back (because women don't need as much food, he insisted).

In Pondicherry, one gorgeous moonlit night after a romantic French meal (that I paid for), he outcrassed even the average Indian cad. Crawling into my bed, he started stroking and kissing, not unpleasantly, especially as I couldn't see him. He sounded like Russell Crowe (you wouldn't kick HIM out of bed, would ya?). It was easy to pretend. It was all going *swimmingly*. His fingers found their way into places which responded in a distinctly ... shall we say gushy manner? He was surprisingly dexterous and I was readier than I'd thought. When he suddenly reached past me to the bedside table and rummaged in its drawer (instead of in mine, which is what he should've carried on doing), there was a clang against wood and a click around my wrists. Something fluffy but also metallic wrapped itself round them.

Shaken out of my nearly-there glow, I gaped for a minute, then yelped, jumping out of bed and half-way across the room at the same time. He shushed me angrily, flicking the light on at the same time. In the naked light of the hostel room, I found a pair of fluffy pink handcuffs clamped around my trembling wrists.

'What the hell is that?' I screamed. 'I bought it just for you,' he said petulantly. 'I got extra-small ones because you have tiny wrists.' Tiny wrists. Was my tiny brain as obvious? I had to have one to be with this guy. 'Take it off,' I insisted, 'take it off NOW!' After observing the floor for what seemed like eternity, he lumbered across to unlock them. Then with a (crocodile?) tear streaking his baby-pink (and suitably podgy) cheek, he told me he did it for me, to spice up my boring Indian life. He had handpicked them too, making sure of not just the size but also colour, to enhance my chocolatey skin. I nearly shed a tear myself, he laid the pathos on so thick, but just as I opened my mouth to soothe and reassure, I heard loud snoring from his bed. He had fallen asleep halfway through patching up.

After which, I travelled to Kathmandu with him. You may well ask why. I couldn't really tell you except that I was still hoping he'd go back to being the man I once (thought I) knew. And I could return to Kolkata triumphantly involved with a guy worth my while.

So here I was. Me still looking out the window. Him, still pushing. Pushing harder. He was determined to crack it now. Literally. And it hurt like the dickens. Was it meant to hurt as much? That's another thing nobody tells you. Did your mother ever sit you down to talk about it? Mine didn't (though I think she would have if I had asked). I attempted to discuss it with my gynae who looked at me like I was filth and I dropped the subject. And that was that.

Although it's going to happen to most of us, is generally painful and always emotionally complex, we still have to go into it blind, trusting men we sometimes barely know to be gentle and sensitive. Let's be honest though, the average guy is not socialized to be sensitive. But then, no one *is* being honest. Not the sugary chick flicks and chick lit that tell us it'll be the most glorious experience of our lives, marked by angels singing and stars linking up in celestial daisy chains to reflect the perfection of that moment. Balderdash and hogwash.

It often isn't even dirty, squishy and good, in a gooey sort of way. But we wouldn't expect that either because Video Library Uncle never, ever let us even have a peep at the shelf of 'grown-up' movies. Not even when we were twenty-three, though the neighbourhood boys had access to it at half that age. He considered it his duty to keep the girls in the *para* pure.

The hymen is like a personal and rather intimately placed Video Library Uncle for every girl. They keep us pure. Apparently. Back when there were no paternity tests, it was one way for a man to know that the children he was bringing up (or not, as it happens with so many men) were indubitably his own. If the woman had her hymen intact when he married her, chances were the children that followed soon after were his.

Later on, of course, there was no way of telling if a woman had been unfaithful except that as she was always tethered to her home like a goat, she was unlikely to have strayed. Nowadays, there isn't any need for a hymen with easy-does-it paternity tests available. It's as superfluous as an appendix, but the world puts its worth at much more. Women have even been known to have it reattached through an expensive and painful operation. Although why would any woman put herself through it when it is of no conceivable use to her? Does she remember the pain of its tearing fondly? Or does she just want to please men. Again.

Men and hymen, that tight little twosome (not men and women, mind). They want it intact because it helps them control women's sexuality and reproduction, but it goes beyond that. The humble pussy plug helps men constrain women socially and economically too. In some Asian countries like Indonesia, women are still tested for their virginity before they are allowed to hold certain posts. Jaw-droppingly anachronistic! There isn't a job in the world for which you need to be a virgin. Not even that of wife.

And we never demand such 'purity' from men. Imagine if we did? If we made them queue up and drop their pants for a painful probing of their private parts, looking for signs of transgression before we gave them a *crack* at a job unrelated to their sexual status (as all jobs are). Imagine the furore. But who's bothered about women routinely violated in that manner? No one.

Rape victims were tested for virginity too till very recently in India. Did they need another strange man ramming unsolicited body parts in? And how can you tell if a woman's been raped by sticking your finger inside her like it's the Thermometer of Truth? All it is, is the opportunity for sad bastards to cop a sordid feel while humiliating the woman for having the nerve to complain. Because which part of not having a hymen suggests you're lying about rape? A missing hymen doesn't indicate sexual experience and not only the virginal get raped!

A number of women are born without a hymen. Up to 15 per cent according to some sources. It can be torn or displaced in the course of vigorous *non-sexual* activity too. I could easily have lost it to a mountain pony in Nainital. I wish I had. It would have been less painful. And what a corking conversation-opener it would have been too. 'I lost my maidenhead on a mountain. To a horse ...' Looking dreamily into the distance like I was recalling an assignation with a centaur and not a mangy pony. I had indeed almost lost it to a horse when mercilessly jogged up mountain paths by a recalcitrant pony on a summer break in my early twenties. But alas, he had been a poor finisher and I was left with not a single story about bestiality for this book.

This little piece of membrane is important to men in yet more ways. The concept of an untouched woman seems to excite them sexually. Experienced women are better in bed, yet men like their women barely legal. Are men wired to feel this way? At one time, it was crucial that a woman be young to have healthy babies, and lots of them. But not now. So why do so many men still demand it? Why do suicide bombers get lured into committing mass murder with the promise of 700 virgins waiting for them in heaven when a handful of MILFs could show them a better time on Earth? Is it virility that's proven in the popping? But you can prove paternity *and* virility without ever needing to pop a cherry. In fact, you can demonstrate it far better if you are making love to a receptive, happy, experienced woman who will tell you exactly where to go (i.e., not to hell, for a change).

Did *I* get what I wanted in the little room at the top of the world? I had imagined my first time to be a thing of beauty and passion. With someone I loved. It didn't work out that way. At the beginning of my odyssey with Duncan I thought I loved him and that it was returned. By the time we got to that hotel room in Kathmandu, I knew neither to be true. I should have walked away, but I was exhausted. By the time I was in my early twenties, I was deathly tired of men and romance and the pressures put on young women by society. I couldn't see anything brighter lighting up my horizon, so I went through with it.

How was I to know that eight years and a couple of men later, the right man would come along after all? I had neither crystal ball nor patience. I just wanted it over with. And all I remember of it now is the awkwardness followed by the ickiness and then the pain. After what felt like an eternity of fumbling, heaving and ramming, with a sharp stab of pain, it was done. Then I lay there disappointed, more disappointed than I had imagined possible. But he had sloped off to wash the blood off his cock. The prick had gone to clean his dick, and I was glad to be alone. Though my thoughts were as awkward a bedfellow as he had been. But then he was back, looking awfully satisfied with himself, and I almost expected him to whip off the bloodstained bedsheet and take it for a round in the lobby like Leon Uris's Arabs. 'Now wasn't that good?' he beamed at me.

Kathmandu was the end of the road for us. I took the next flight home. A few weeks later, he called from Auckland and I told him it was over. He was miffed, but that's as far as it went. He was SO not The One. But to all those who condemn women like me who go looking for the perfect man rather than settle for the one foisted on them (overtly or otherwise), to those who tut when we get it wrong, I say: how was I to know? When did you ever talk to me about it?

3

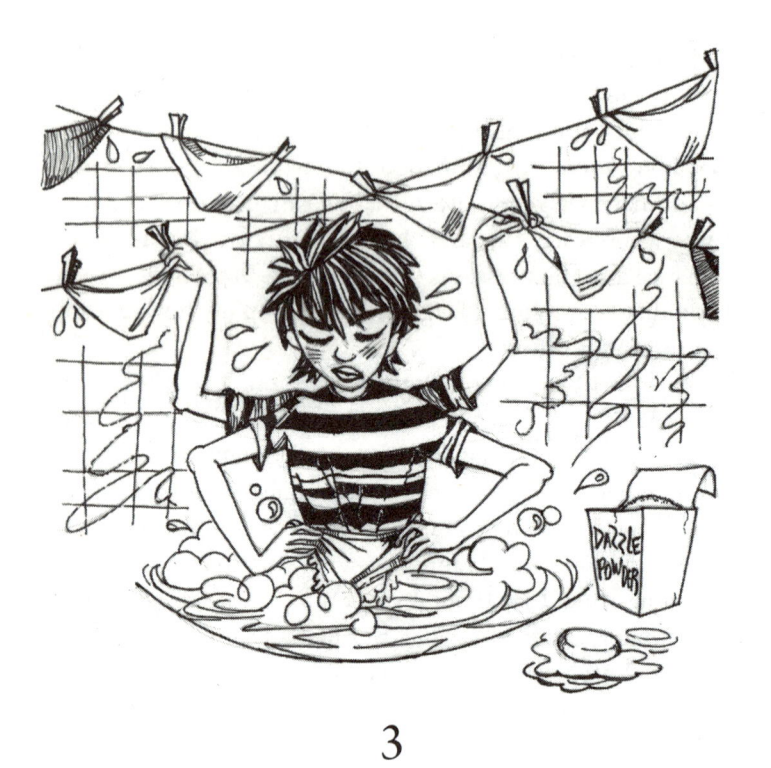

Crimson Tide

'We must talk about it,' said my mother at the onset of my periods in Kolkata. What she didn't know was that this was the *second* month of periods I was experiencing. I had already been through the shock, discomfort and shame, and now felt like a battle-scarred veteran. So I said to her, 'No, no, I already know everything.'

I felt like I did. I had started bleeding the month before, in Bangkok, on our way back from the Philippines. We had lived in the latter for six salubrious years before political upheavals persuaded my father we should return to India. On the way back, we spent a week with that unique entity that Indians call 'family friends'. Friends of someone in the extended family, though no one quite knows whom.

And so my periods began, like almost everything important in my life, far from home. Worse, it started in a sparkling Bangkok apartment full of boys (OK, two, but you know how boys fill space) who wouldn't know a menstrual cycle from a menopausal fug. To be honest, I didn't either! The momentous week it happened, I was as clueless as the young men who uncomfortably shared my space (uncomfortable for *me*, they didn't even know something was up. Or down. Terrifyingly trickling down).

I was only eleven. It had come two *years* before I was warned it would. If my mother had already told me about it, as she claims she did, I couldn't remember a word of it when it happened. I was terrified. Was that poo streaking my pants? Was it blood? Was I dirty or diseased or both? Could I stop it, or at least hide it? Worse even than staining their radiant upholstery and sheets would be keeling over and dying from blood loss. How embarrassing would that be for my parents?

'We are banned from all our friends' homes, Dita, because *your* daughter sullied the spotless satin sheets of the last one wherein we stayed. We can no longer hold our heads up high. Worse, we can never go on holiday again,' I imagined my father saying. To which my mother might have responded, 'It was decidedly thoughtless of *your* daughter to besmirch their sheets so but there are always hotels. Specially the kind that have those rich, dark sheets and Gothic furniture. Gold taps and ornate mirrors in the bathroom. Stains don't show up easily at such places.' Sounds of choking followed by a spluttered, 'Holiday in a hotel? Never! That is not what I was brought up to do. Good Indian travellers always stay with friends, no matter how tenuous the connection. It is the Gandhian thing to do.'

This conversation never happened because dialogue between my parents was not only limited at that stage in their marriage, it was not scripted by a Victorian ha'penny novelist either. But if my father had ever discussed his holiday philosophy, that would have been the gist of it. To be fair to my parents, whatever their holiday philosophy, had they known what was going on, I might have been scolded as always, but then, they would have helped. Both of them.

However, I couldn't find the courage to tell them and here we were. Guests in an impossibly posh apartment. And I was bleeding for the first time. Like everything else in my life, my period had chosen the most awkward moment to make its appearance. Or perhaps it was an early lesson in mucking through (with the emphasis firmly on muck), at which I became amazingly adept as I went along.

We were on a final journey home after all those years, and my heart was breaking. Can a breaking heart cause the premature cracking of eggs? Who knows? What I did know was that I didn't want to go back to Kolkata. With my beloved great grandfather gone to the Big Library in the Sky, Kolkata held very little appeal for me. On our holidays there while we were based in Manila, I had been overwhelmed by the heat, dust and din. I found people too censorious and intrusive, and they did not take to me in turn. And where were the blue skies and wide open spaces I'd grown to love in the Philippines?

But to Kolkata we headed because that's what Baba deemed best. Little did I know what else was in store. Already worried about making a fool of myself (I was at that age when I did it effortlessly and often) in a house full of strangers, I felt distinctly funny through dinner that first night, delicious though the meal of coconut chicken with fragrant rice was. And it wasn't my usual discomfiture with cutlery causing it. Going to bed in a strangely silent house where the older, rather nice-looking boy talked not at all, I woke in the early hours with horrific stomach cramps and something oozing stickily from between my legs. I stumbled to the bathroom, mumbling my thanks to the God of Brief Things that they had contained it in my pretty pastel ones, touching the shimmering sheets not at all. In the pristine bathroom on the landing, I anxiously peeked inside them to find streaks of gelatinous crimson clinging to my suddenly not-so-little-girl parts. The coconutty chicken from earlier threatened to make a reappearance. But no. Throwing up would be completely the wrong thing to do.

Minimize the mess, not create more! I scolded myself in a frightened whisper. Stealthily filling the bath with cold water, I dumped some soap in it, and quietly got in so as not to alert anyone. Then with greater guilt than Goebbels ever knew, I washed myself and my underpants. I hung them up where I hoped they would not be detected. Still damp and more terrified than ever, I stuffed several minute schoolgirl handkerchiefs down a pair of fresh pants to catch the blood (fortunately scant) and slid back into bed.

That was just the start. In that one week of summer, I would know more underhand underpant washing and petrifying worry and shame than ever before. I nearly got found out too. While everyone watched Mel Brook's *To Be or Not to Be*, I attempted to sneak out to do my hourly washing up. I had almost reached the bathroom at the end of their gleaming corridor when Boy Who Talks Rarely But Always Looks Godlike turned up. 'Is everything OK?' he asked quietly. In my eleven-year-old head, it morphed into an interrogation. I quaked. 'To the bedroom. Yes, bedroom. I was heading for the bedroom,' I waffled, pointing vaguely in the direction of the kitchen.

His brows furrowed in what was clearly suspicion (though looking back, it so easily could have been concern for his half-wit guest). Why couldn't I have just said 'bathroom', I cringed inwardly. After all, people do perfectly innocent things in bathrooms too. 'But your bedroom is that way.' 'Oh!' I jumped as if shot, colouring guiltily. I rushed to my bedroom with my ears burning in embarrassment, coughing out choked thank yous as I went. And there I stayed feigning sleep till the house retired for the night and I could conduct my ablutions in peace.

What got me through that desperately difficult week was that I wasn't bleeding heavily. And that, as always, my parents were completely oblivious to my predicament. The previous year, it had taken them months to realize I had lost my braces in a camping trip. I had gone camping with my class with the biggest, shiniest braces anyone had ever seen. But they weren't clamped to my teeth. They were the kind you removed at night, and so I did. In the morning while upping sticks, I left my smelly little box of dental tricks behind. By the time I realized what had happened, there was no way I could go back to retrieve it. For months after, I pretended I still had it. On the odd occasion I was asked about them, I would claim I was just about to put them on. It worked because they really weren't in the business of looking at me much.

Till something made them suspicious and they asked to see the braces. I confessed I had lost them and all hell broke loose for about half an hour, until they found something else to fret about. My teeth never got straightened and I, for the most part, have not had cause to regret it except when the particularly gauche or deliberately mean have pointed it out. Or the ridiculously young who can't help but point out the obvious. Like the little brother of Godlike Boy Who Only Spoke Once. He asked me shyly about my teeth in the course of that eventful trip.

'Your teeth are funny,' he giggled across the table from me at dinner one night. 'They want to do a silly stroll when they're being told to walk properly.' I smiled in relief. Talking about teeth doing silly things was easier than worrying about girl parts doing upsetting things. 'They are a little rebellious,' I grinned at him. 'A bit like your hair, standing up like that,' I said, but without hurtful intent.

He smoothed it down sheepishly with the same hand that had been in his rice. I could then see why his hair stood on end. 'Yeah,' he whispered, 'I'm stuck with it.' I smothered a laugh, knowing it wouldn't be a problem when he grew up (and stopped sticking food in his hair). 'Me too,' I said. Then he confided, 'Nobody else knows my hair stands up because it's really antennae. I get messages from aliens through them.' I nodded seriously, 'It's the same with me. I distract people with my gnashers. While they're looking at my teeth, I slip away on top secret missions.' We bumped fists. 'This conversation never happened,' he said, and turned away to dig into his rice.

Just like that conversation never happened, periods are treated like they don't exist. Or if they do, it's seen as such a vile, unnatural, almost criminal act that a culture of shamed silence has grown up around it. Really, people, a woman bleeding so she can ensure the survival of the human race, YOUR survival, needs to be punished, banished and confined? Even in liberal Indian homes, talking about it in the presence of men remains taboo. On our return to India, it was made clear to me that though I could say pretty much what I wanted to my parents, there was a slew of subjects, including periods (especially periods), that should never be mentioned outside the home. But I have to confess I have lapsed time and again, usually deliberately, because I've never understood the need to shield men from this most natural of processes.

Girls are told so little that many think they are dying when it happens the first time. Even those who have had a sketchy talk are shocked (the clue's in 'sketchy'). And everyone else must be spared discussion about it too.

An Instagram image went viral not so long ago. Instead of the regulation kittens, babies or semi-clad women, it featured a supine, fully clothed woman with a dark, barely discernible bloodstain on her grey track pants, like women often get when sleeping. Yet, this caused such a storm of shock, horror and revulsion that the picture was taken off the site. Yes, in this day and age, when no one bats an eyelid at the most depraved images of violence or sex, a woman menstruating creates a controversy. Evidently, we are expected to continue treating it like a dirty secret.

Rupi Kaur, who had posted the picture to protest just that approach to menstruation, hit back saying, 'Instagram, you deleted my photo twice, stating it goes against community guidelines. I will not apologize for not feeding the ego and pride of a misogynist society that will have my body in underwear but not be okay with a small leak[8].' Similarly, Kiran Gandhi ran the London Marathon recently with menstrual blood streaming down her legs, to some praise and not unexpectedly, a lot of flak. The gutsy young lady responded, 'Culture is happy to speak about and objectify the parts of the body that can be sexually consumed by others, but the moment we talk about something that's not for the enjoyment of others, like a period, everyone becomes deeply uncomfortable. I ran with blood dripping down my legs to say it does exist, and we overcome it every day[9].'

Al Capone may be dead and gone but Omerta lives and affects the everyday lives of ordinary women. And those appalling euphemisms – that time of the month, having the blob on, jam rags – don't they do the same job of insisting it's so terrible it should not be named (like Voldemort but worse)? I can't casually drop it into conversation even though I can discuss disease (and this is *not* a disease, no matter what your mausi tells you) in great, gruesome detail? Why does that not horrify you like the mere mention of my utterly normal, completely harmless (to you) periods do?

This subject remains off-limits in the West as well. You might mention it to another woman when explaining your mood or the extra trips to the loo, but that too would have to be accompanied by some coy beating about the bush. Hannah Betts in *The Telegraph* says it doesn't matter where in the world you live, 'Menstruation constitutes the great, shared silence at the heart of female existence', and 'I've been bleeding for 30-plus years, with a variety of ever-evolving symptoms from passing out via great tranches of pain to glassy, lobotomised exhaustion. Yet I'm not supposed to talk about it. It's a vast part of my life, and the lives of those around me that society expects to go entirely unspoken.'[10]

If periods are a naughty thing that women do *just because*, then it stands to reason that no sympathy is spared for our pain and discomfort. Research by the British National Health Service suggests 90 per cent of *all* women experience period pain. Of that percentage, 14 per cent of women are regularly incapacitated by the severity of the pain. But these are 'women's problems' – insignificant, almost unbelievable and most certainly, ridiculous. It's never a real reason to shirk our responsibilities.

Within a few months of the start of my periods, a pattern was set. Leading up to the bleeding, I would get the most excruciating cramps. And then for seven days out of a month, I bled such quantities that it seemed almost impossible there would be blood left in my tiny frame after. I learnt to cope. But just when I thought I'd got to grips with the worst, the fainting started. The sight of my blood didn't make me swoon. Women are rarely affected by that, as if by design. After all, they may have the gore of childbirth to deal with one day. No, it was the hideous pain. Reeling with pain, I would get up to deal with it. Minutes later, I would find myself lying on a cold floor with a vague recollection of the rush of darkness that had overtaken me, and a bruised and aching face to add to the agony I was already in.

Drama became a menstrual staple for me, but as a family, we learnt to laugh about it the year my younger sister started hers. Our periods would often begin together. Bleeding at the same time wasn't unusual but one fine day, we found ourselves fainting in unison too. Every time I passed out, my sister followed suit, which was especially ironic in siblings not especially close. Bizarrely, it made our periods more bearable because it was comic, and gave us the giggles, even if it meant we now had bruises and our mother's perpetual hovering to deal with as well. We called it the Sen Sisters' Synchronized Swooning, and said we'd take it on the road, though we never did.

Despite all that, our lot's been pretty cushy compared to what poor women endure the world over. 'One in three women worldwide,' say the World Toilet People, 'risk shame, disease, harassment and even attack because they have nowhere safe to change and clean themselves when menstruating. In many countries, girls have no option but to stay home[11].'

But many girls aren't even allowed to stay home! They are sent out to change and sleep in filthy cowsheds and other unimaginably unhygienic places, imperilling the reproductive health they are prized for (the only thing they are prized for). In our oh-so-mahaan Bharat, women in underprivileged or traditional homes aren't allowed to cook, preserve pickles, set curd or water the plants while bleeding (a blessed relief). But contact with men and even women, including family members who might help them through it, is also forbidden, for fear they will 'infect' those around them. So they are also excluded from all social occasions and the temple. And in the mother of all ironies, they are even barred from entering the temple of the Menstruating Goddess herself, Kamyakha Devi, in the hills of Assam! Of course, menstruating women have been banned from entering places of worship for thousands of years. Not much has changed since the Bible pronounced, 'If her issue be blood, she shall be put apart seven days: and whosoever toucheth her shall be unclean. And everything she lieth upon shall be unclean.' Not only have they not stopped reminding us of this (yawn), every major religion and their adherents continue to enforce these rigours on bleeding women, with punishments for the smallest lapses.

Why do they do it? Miranda Farage in her book, *The Vulva*, suggests men lash out against menstruating women out of fear. 'As bleeding is a sign of injury, our ancestors may have viewed cyclical bleeding – without dying – as a supernatural event'. [12] And the supernatural is not only scary but worth guarding against.

While the ignorant will insist that the constraints placed on menstruating women are a means to safeguard other people's health, the more sophisticated have convinced themselves that it's about propriety and privacy because women are so easily embarrassed. Blushing and swooning at the mere mention of menses is what women do, right? Wrong. They do that from pain and blood loss.

So what is it really that impels men (and the many, many women who toe the patriarchal line, often gleefully) to punish menstruating women? Is it fear, embarrassment or the belief they are doing it for our good (like rape, beatings, FGM)? Patriarchal society penalizes women for being women in the same way they muzzle and marginalize people of different sexual orientations and colour. We are a threat because we are different. We have different priorities and compulsions. We can, if given an inch, upset the very fabric of the society they have had to bludgeon so many to stitch together.

So, they are being canny when they keep us down for improbable reasons like our infectious menstrual blood but they are also genuinely scared. Frightened of losing their foothold at the top of the heap of all those they have dispossessed and subjugated. Now that's proper scary stuff. But it's funny too. The 'I don't know whether to laugh or cry' kinda funny. For example, contact with menstruating women is supposed to ruin creatures as diverse as pigs and men (maybe not so different after all)! Men fall ill and bacon rots (and neither is true as I've tested both). Yet the British Medical Journal was sure of it as late as 1878.

School walls, books and the brains of others must also rot in contact with menstrual blood. How else can you explain the abysmal ignorance all around? Or why in some countries women are prohibited from entering educational institutions when bleeding. Not long ago in Nepal, Hindu leaders banned menstruating women from entering schools, threatening them with expulsion from their villages if they did. Back in Swachh Bharat, urban schools have filthy toilets, and in the villages, there are no toilets at all. Concentrating on lessons is hard enough for a girl getting to grips with this new and traumatic bodily process, without having no place to change or dispose of period paraphernalia. Continuing with their education is made so difficult for these young women that 23 per cent of them leave for menial jobs and arranged marriages.

That's when it stops being a 'woman's issue' (it issues from us, but it never was just our problem). When women are denied education, the whole world suffers with them, whether they realize it or not. Educated women are healthier, have smaller families, earn more, positively impacting on development. So money, the concept even the most ignorant bigot understands, slips through their fingers because they won't treat girls transitioning into womanhood with the consideration the latter require to make that leap.

That's not to say there aren't laudable campaigns trying to address the issue. Inspired by the actions of a woman artist in Germany, female students at Jamia Millia Islamia and the University of Delhi stuck sanitary napkins with anti-sexist slogans in and around their institutions in 2015. It may have done nothing but shock, but shocking people into some sense is long overdue. There are also activists (some of them men!) trying to make the monthly bleed more hygienic and less uncomfortable for underprivileged women. 70 per cent of Indian women are prey to reproductive diseases because they are too poor to afford sanitary napkins and use dirty rags instead.

Murugunantham from Tamil Nadu is a knight in shining sanitary towel. He actually wore pads to understand the menstruating woman's predicament better. He saw that his wife, like most poor women, was forced to use filthy, threadbare scraps to contain the flow, though they caused frequent infections. He decided to look into this thing he knew absolutely nothing about, although it was clearly happening all around him regularly. He not only tried sanitary towels out on himself, he also walked around wearing a pretend-uterus, a football bladder filled with goat's blood from a butcher. He even studied used sanitary pads. All of which, predictably, led to first his village and then his own family shunning him. But Murugunantham carried on despite their desertion and built a simple but effective machine that made affordable pads for the millions of women who needed them. His machine has now gone global and his village, friends and family have welcomed him back, hailing him as the hero he always was.[13]

Similarly, Dhirendra Pratap Singh and Ameet Mehta help the Uttar Pradesh government build schools with clean toilets for girls, enabling them to continue their education even after their menses start[14]. *My* period hero is my Dad. Yes, that guy with the horrible holiday philosophy. But he had the best possible approach to bringing up his daughters where it really mattered. Unlike the reported 50 per cent of Indian men who never buy sanitary napkins for their female relatives, sending these aching, oozing women out to do it themselves, Baba would march out every time we had our periods to get us everything we needed to be clean and comfortable. We could also always talk to him about it without reservations. It made such a difference to our lives, even if he didn't change the world with what he did. Or did he? By assuring us, 'We'll look after everything else, so you can just skip to the loo, my darlings', and following it through, he sprang two more bright, independent and determined women on the world. And when it comes to that kind of woman, *or man*, the more the merrier, you know.

As that first flow of blood staunched, my visit to Bangkok

became happier. The little chat at the table had something to do with it too. Someone had understood and empathized with my discomfort even if they hadn't known its nature. With the illicit washing and fear of discovery behind me, I began to take an interest in my colourful surroundings. My sketchbook filled up with the stylized mythical monsters that stood guard at the Grand Palace. I found a kind of peace at the Wat Pho, temple of the Reclining Buddha, an acceptance that one chapter of my life was over and another about to begin. And it may even be bearable. After all, I'd just survived a week of bleeding, another new and unexpected interloper.

When I had my second round in Kolkata, Ma helped me understand the hows and whens, despite my protestations that I already knew everything about it. She explained that it was neither dirt nor disease and would certainly not lead to my untimely demise. Like our return to Kolkata, it was a new beginning – the beginning of womanhood for me, and that couldn't be bad. But history has a way of repeating itself. Twenty-eight years later, I found myself bleeding in a most perplexing way again.

This time, it did not herald a new life.

4

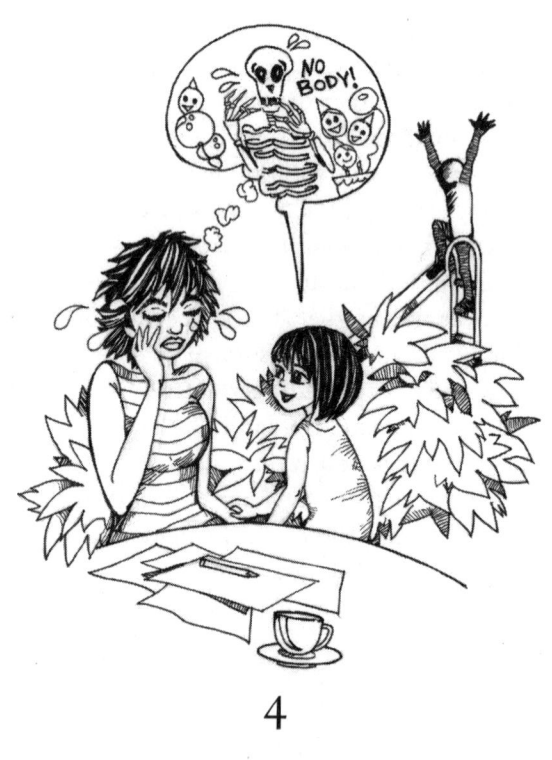

May Day, May Day

Everyone claims it happens to them. But that morning, I really did wake up with a sense of foreboding. Is it my fortieth birthday already, I wondered woozily. No it wasn't, the glowing date on my bedside clock assured me. It was still several months away and though I was disturbed by its approach, why did this day of all days feel so wrong?

Switching on the computer after dropping both kids off at school, I felt strangely unsettled. Tick tock went the hallway clock sotto voce, as if warning me of something so terrible that it didn't dare say it aloud. In our happy home of eight years, there was a tangible air of doom. Doom not gloom, on this rare sparklingly bright day in Sherwood Forest where we lived. I knew the difference. Gloom I suffered from often. This uneasiness was physical. Like a storm brewing inside me. I started work tentatively. Writhing in discomfort every now and then.

The locus of the looming disaster seemed to be in my stomach. Typing standing up might help, I thought. But stand still I could not. I shifted from leg to leg as if it were an age-old antidote against doom. It wasn't, to my knowledge, even an antidote against age, or our ageing celebrities would have turned it into a health fad a long time ago.

Thoughts of divas inevitably led me to check into Facebook. It greeted me with the usual faux jovial, 'So what's on your mind today?' I'm not sure, I thought. How strange, how unlike me. And how totally not suitable for an update, which requires an assurance beyond the realms of reality. An update that confessed to uncertainty and uneasiness would simply get trampled in the rush of dazzlingly decorated cakes concocted from scratch, promotions that happen on the hour and flawlessly crafted origami butterflies made in fifteen seconds flat. And who can compete with the attractions of Mrs Perfect's perfectly turned out tween who's brought home the inter-school Miss Never-puts-a-foot-wrong corsage AGAIN?

'I have no triumphs to offer you today, but stick with me won't you, Facebook?' I whispered to the screen, wondering yet again what could be troubling me on such a fine day. Something that wasn't creeping up on me, it turned out, so much as creeping down my leg. A warm trickle, out of nowhere, was making tracks down my inner thigh. I tried wishing it away (washing it away would have been the sensible option but sensible isn't something I do). Whatever it was, I wanted it to stop. I wanted it to snake back into me, back where it belonged. Humming Joe Cocker to help it along didn't work either. So, using the 'a watched kettle never boils' principle, I ignored it instead, focusing on a new Facebook friend who had been persistently making inroads into my life for about a week, clearly keen to get to know me.

'You are such a special woman,' he was saying. He's spotted that already? My wry amusement turned to surprise as warmth flooded my tummy. But it wasn't the warmth of gratification. That little knot of unease I'd had all morning in my stomach, tight as an egg, felt like it had cracked open. Something was seeping out with a sigh of relief, but also despondency. Hoping the trickle was just the usual, just a bit early, I sat down and crossed my legs, attempting to hold it in, putting off the inevitable dash to clean up. I was resisting even looking at it. But it evidently had no intention of being anything quite so innocuous as 'just the usual'. From trickle to sludge to a steady crimson tide, it soon had all my attention.

I watched with disbelief as it slid down my legs, gluing my beige cotton trousers to me and pooling on the butcher's blue carpet at my feet. Pushing away the pinpricks of pain that had just begun to make themselves felt, I was transfixed as well as baffled by what was happening. On the screen in the meantime, quite without preamble, the man had launched into a description of what he would do to me on his office desk.

'Lying you down, I'd sling your legs around my neck so I can sink my face into your honeypot.' Honeypot?? You might be in for a surprise, I thought distractedly. SO not full of honey today. 'Then inserting my tongue into you, I shall lap at your sugar walls lasciviously.' Ooh, I thought, what big words you know, Grandad. 'I shall lick you till you're writhing, pinioned on my tongue. And you will shudder to the most monumental climax.'

I *am* shuddering but not from excitement, I thought queasily as I looked down at my spattered crotch. Soaked through with a rusty, jellied blood that's the furthest thing from cum. Nor could I shake off the horrific vision of his face going splat on my twat. There are indeed times when you don't want a man going down on you though it isn't often. Fleetingly, I heard disgruntled men everywhere, throwing their hands up in exasperation as they exclaimed, 'But how do we know when?' When we're haemorrhaging on our living room floor, for example. Like about now. And as irascible as the unfolding drama was making me feel, I couldn't pin it on the man cyber-tonguing me from the other end of the world, much as I wanted to. Or on *any* man. I was much too busy bleeding anyway. My stomach lurched once again, expelling more gore. Retching, I took a tremulous step away from the spreading stain at my feet, meaning to make my way to the sterile safe haven of the bathroom. But suddenly I was overwhelmed by a pain so invasive, so much like the wrenching labour spasms I experienced with my first baby that I didn't have to wonder any more. Suddenly I knew. Suddenly my uppermost thought was no longer the unwelcome sexual turn the chat had taken, bloodied carpet or persistent pain. It was grief. I had just lost a baby, a baby I didn't know I had. A little one I would never get to gaze at, hold or name. An infant I didn't even get to savour the thought of. As the full force of my loss struck me, so did another wave of pain.

I passed out.

***

Two days later, ensconced in bed, warmed by the gentle English sunlight streaming through the window and even gentler care from my husband, I found the courage to face the world again, if only the virtual world. 'How are you this fine and dandy morning?' Facebook cackled raucously in my face as I logged in. And though the sensible part of my psyche screamed (OK, the sensible me neither screams nor ever gets heard) – shut it down, shut it down NOW, I didn't. Instead I found myself telling the world how I felt. 'An endlessly aching void has opened up inside me ...'

It felt like a bottomless grief, a pain I would never see the back of. A spring of a few ups and downs, perhaps a handful more than usual, had led to this – the most searing summer I have lived through. In the long, hot summer of '83, thirty years before this one, Bananarama had crooned about the 'crool, crool summer' their mullet-headed, kerchief-necked ('twas the eighties, after all) lover left them. Several things rather essential to happiness left me that summer: my mystery baby, my hard-won peace of mind, but worst of all, my senses, mysteriously sidling away just when I needed them most.

'No One Puts Baby in the Corner'

Remember Patrick Swayze squaring up to Jennifer Grey's celluloid tormentors with that line in *Dirty Dancing*? But Patrick (or St Paddy, patron saint of babies-in-corners as he's now known) couldn't have stopped the harrowing loss of Baby that mild, summer morning. Factors beyond his control and more importantly, mine, decided what happened to my little-one-to-be. Baby could not have been more than six weeks old, unformed, and most of all, unknown, *even* to me. My first phone call, two days later, confirmed what I had gut-wrenchingly, heartbreakingly suspected. There was almost no doubt it was a miscarriage. They couldn't be absolutely sure at such an early stage, they said, but my halting description of the events of that fateful morning matched everything they knew about it. When I finally put the phone down, I was wiser but no happier.

Paddy was wrong. Your own body can and will put Baby in a corner, a distant, no-longer-of-this-world corner, if the conditions aren't right. And they so often aren't. 20 per cent of all pregnancies fail, with 85 per cent of these sudden cessations occurring in the first twelve weeks. Like me, many women who miscarry early aren't even aware they were pregnant. Not having known doesn't help in the least. If anything, there's an extra bit of guilt to be found in that. And all the scientific debunking in the world doesn't make a dent in it. Not to the bereaved mother or the people in her life her who would pin it on her. I blamed myself squarely. Not only had I been unaware of its existence, I hadn't really wanted one at that stage of my life. Had I wished it away? Could I have looked after myself and therefore, Baby, better? Was I at fault after all?

Unlike many women in my situation, I was lucky to have nothing to fear from anyone else. In India, there is a higher incidence of both 'gendercide' and miscarriage than in the rest of the world. Of the 309,546 crimes against women reported in 2013, 118,866 were domestic in nature. Considering that Indian women are also, allegedly, 20 per cent more likely to suffer miscarriages, it follows that women losing a baby, especially a boy baby in India, can expect a backlash. I didn't, my husband and family had nothing but support for me, but I still needed answers.

Awright Google, I said to the all-knowing modern Oracle in that now-prescribed jaunty tone with which it must be approached, how did my baby ... die? I faltered over the word that sent my spirits plummeting to lows I hadn't known existed. Google cast its gimlet eye over the causes of early miscarriages, laconically laying them out before me. Early miscarriages typically take place because the embryo isn't evolving as it should. This arrested development is usually caused by malfunctioning chromosomes, which affect as many as three-quarters of all fertilized eggs in the early stages of pregnancy. And for no known reason.

So, Baby stops growing. Then Baby dies.

Baby or Bust

But no one is to blame, it was drummed home again. Yet you can drum all you want and it may not register, because which woman hasn't grown up with the weight of the world on her shoulders? Everything from Original Sin (don't get me started) to social disorder and natural disasters are our fault. And when it comes to All Things Baby, there are no two ways about it. As South African president Jacob Zuma reminded women in 2012, 'Daughters who are not getting married is a problem in society. That's a distortion. You've got to have kids. Kids are important to a woman because they give extra training to be a woman[15].'

It wasn't only South African society that was in peril from women who couldn't or wouldn't reproduce on demand. 'I would like to tell all my Hindu mothers and sisters that if they don't have five children, there will be no balance in India in the future', warned the BJP's Shyamal Goswami[16]. When we do have children (for *ourselves* and not to please these goons), we continue to be held accountable for the sex of our offspring when the world knows for a FACT now that the father's chromosomes decide gender.

You see, gender in humans is governed by a couple of sex

chromosomes called gonosomes. Women have two of the same (XX) while men have one of each type (XY). Whether Baby is male or female depends ENTIRELY on the chromosome X or Y received from Dad. Could this *be* any clearer (said à la Chandler, as it must)? Clearly not clear to some, as patriarchs and old wives plough on with their prejudices regardless. Not just to do with gender but with healthy foetal growth as well.

'Her unreliable woman's body is to blame,' they mutter menacingly. 'Couldn't she have grown strong chromosomes? She had no trouble sprouting breasts (shameless hussy)!' 'How is it even possible,' they carry on venomously, 'that a mother loses a life growing inside her and it's not her fault?'

That, of course, is a rhetorical question. Convinced as they are that the woman is at fault, these barren/irresponsible/inept women are then banished/punished/murdered. After all, why have a woman hang around if she can't reproduce? According to the Indian Crimes Records Bureau, a bride is killed every hour in India. They are killed for a multitude of reasons including their sometimes pernicious inability to produce a baby. Yet, in 50 per cent of such cases, factors to do with the father are responsible for the loss. 'What's that,' the misogynist hordes hiss, 'you aren't suggesting Beta/Poltu is the deficient one, are you?'

Of course I am. Take Kell's Disease for example. A father with the rare Kell antigen in his blood could be behind his partners' many miscarriages. A Kell-positive man can father a healthy first baby. But after that, the antibodies triggered by the Kell factor in the first pregnancy can attack subsequent babies, causing miscarriages and stillbirths.

Henry VIII has now been revealed to be a classic example of the Kell factor wreaking havoc. His six wives and many mistresses put together produced just four live babies between them. Every other pregnancy ended in miscarriage or a stillbirth[17]. Like all other men of his ilk (and women-hating, women-baiting women, of whom there are plenty), he blamed his ladeez for this tragic series of losses. One was divorced as a result, and two beheaded.

Not that different from the average ignoramus who punishes his wife for his own failings in the baby-begetting department. Except that Henry had the excuse of having lived 500 years ago in less enlightened times. And fat, hirsute, and turbaned though he was, isn't it time our desi biraderi found themselves another role model?

Working myself into a bit of a frenzy over these miscarriages of justice was meant to keep my mind off my own loss. But I couldn't stop thinking about it. That it happened so often to so many women didn't make it easier to bear. That I already had two beautiful children and was under no pressure to produce a third, didn't make me feel less disconsolate. My world had come to a shuddering, juddering halt. It was a beautiful time of year in Sherwood Forest, with perfect cotton-puff clouds floating in a startlingly blue sky, and I should have enjoyed it like every year before that. I should have been splashing in the paddling pool with my boisterous young children, telling them stories on our creaky wooden swing as evening drew in, enthusiastically tucking into the grilled pepper steaks and ratatouille that my husband made so well on our wood stove in the garden.

I was doing none of that. But after two days of lying in bed and looking out of the window at the tops of our Robin-Hood-green walnut trees, I knew I had to pull myself together and get on with life. I had two young 'uns who needed me. So I did. But it was a frankly Herculean effort (Or Athenean. Or something. There should be a female word to describe a mammoth task, we do 'em so often). Grief I had known before, though nothing quite like that for a lost child. This was more searing, more relentlessly undermining, more confusing than anything I'd felt before. As I plunged back into everyday life and had those utterly endearing conversations I'd always had with my children, the grief receded. Because, after all, here were my living, breathing babies, as loving and loveable as ever.

'Shall I tell you a joke, Mommy? It will cheer you up,' my three-year-old daughter offered. We were sitting in the sun reading, writing and shelling peas, though that last activity had been largely forgotten. Her five-year-old brother was repeatedly climbing up the slide rather than sliding down it. Every time he got to the top, he looked as proud as Tenzing Norgay on the crest of Everest. He made the necessary cheering noises for his imaginary crowd of admirers, then repeated the whole thing again, keeping himself commendably entertained in this manner.

His sister, seeing my shoulders droop and my mouth turn down at the corners as it did several times a day at the time, ran over to me. I forced a smile as I pulled her close. 'Why did the skeleton go to the party alone?' she asked. Then, more than happy to go straight to the punchline without having to wait for me to hazard a guess, 'because he had no-body!' And I dissolved into tears at the thought of the lonely skeleton, much to my daughter's amazement and my embarrassment and regret ever after. I cried a lot and felt alone often even when surrounded by my beautiful family.

I couldn't understand the grief, nor did I want to give into it, but it felt inexorable. I lived in a fairly isolated place, with little passing traffic, especially of the human kind (squirrels and birdies there were aplenty). My children were spending more time at school than before. And my husband had started a new job, rather unfortunately just before the miscarriage, which kept him away long hours in the day. It was like I had left the kitchen door open and from the depths of the mysterious green that is the heart of Sherwood had come a whistling wind. With it, a gnawing loneliness I should not have felt at all.

It took me months to pick up that phone again and ask the question, 'Why do I feel this way?' (In the UK, most medical conversations are over the phone these days, including the ones that go, 'My heart is hanging out of my rib cage, what should I do?' 'Push it back in firmly,' someone will respond in a bored monotone, 'and then try a spot of gardening. Fresh air will do you no end of good.')

This time, however, I was lucky to be put through to a community counsellor who, having listened to the whole sorry saga starting with my miscarriage, which by then was a few months old, suggested gently that perhaps I wasn't 'at fault'. Perhaps it was post-partum depression. He proffered it as the most likely explanation for a deep depression like mine on the heels of a miscarriage. And there was help to be had. I would have to start by calling my GP. 'Oh,' I muttered to the bewildered man who had expected more enthusiasm. I was grateful he had thrown me a lifeline. I now had a name to my malaise and something to blame for the messes of the previous months, but I did not have a solution. Because I did not intend to go to a doctor with it. To tell you why, I would have to go back more than sixty years to a well-heeled home in Kolkata ...

5

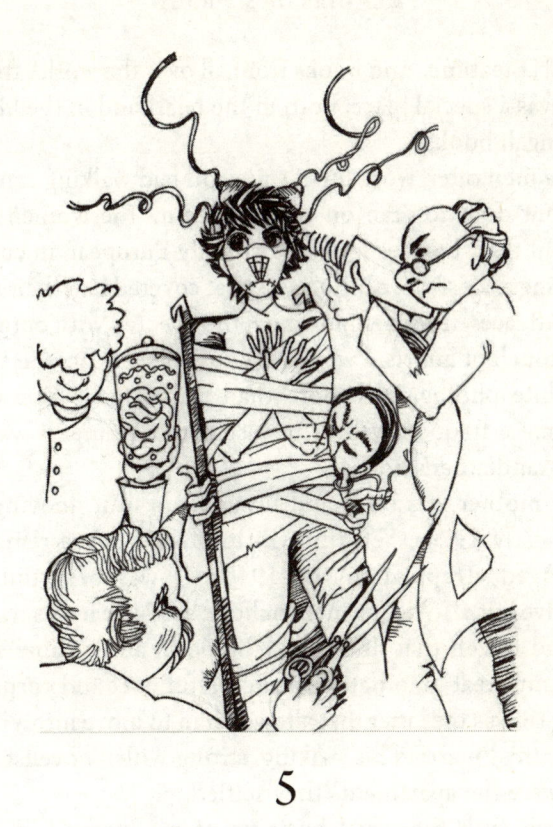

Madness Becomes Her

In the genteel homes of the Bengali intelligentsia of post-WW II Kolkata, you would find proud Chesterfields alongside grandfather clocks in book-choked libraries. They had the space, sometimes the money and always the bibliographical fervour to have whole rooms dedicated to books. With the usual appurtenances: the magnifying glass, the beautifully detailed globe that swung with a creak, the fine china that arrived at teatime. And books from all over the world, though there was a special place, both in the heart and in the library, for Bengali books.

The men often wore linen suits and had walking canes by the front door to grab on their way out. The women wore saris but their blouses looked distinctly European in cut and trimmings. Most wore big glasses that covered half their softly rounded faces, from behind which they peered with optimism and a touch of hubris. I would encounter such faces in black-and-white photographs more than thirty years later when I became a frequent visitor to just such a home. It was my great-grandfather's house.

My mother was born and brought up in it, moving out in the early 1970s. Yet, through it all, the house remained unchanged. Trapped in the 1940s, it was beautiful and evocative but also deeply melancholic, because it was tragedy that had frozen that once-lively home in an icy time warp. When my great-grandfather, a successful poet and corporate bigwig (it was the latter that allowed him to move into a home such as this) married his striking, strong-willed novelist wife, these were the apartments they settled in.

Along with the usual business of producing two well-favoured daughters, they got on with their literary lives, being published and earning acclaim, which came with awards I spied on dusty shelves many years later. They were surrounded by similarly creative souls who got together in their elegant house for food, laughter and inspiration. Poems, novels and the occasional romance were spawned in this sparkling home. The daughters grew up and met men of intellect and charm whom they married, and it was at this point that this story of a family's triumph turned into tragedy.

Their older daughter, Millie, was dazzling, at least to the

outside world. She was bright, beautiful and every bit as talented as her parents. And unlike her quieter sibling, she was vivacious; chattering, chortling and proselytizing, she turned heads as she wafted past in her sweet-smelling cotton saris. Saris which had remained the hallmark of the freedom-fighting Indian, no matter what their position in society. Because though decorative, she was also a deep thinker, and her country's pain was her pain. In fact, she felt intensely and often, but she channelled it into crusades and creative endeavour. And nobody thought the intensity of her pain unusual.

She married a man on the cusp of success. Yet he, like her, was a sensitive soul, more fragile than anyone suspected. Married, in a home of their own for the first time and passionately in love, together they created *hell* on earth. They also created a child, a little girl, the spitting image of her mother, with the promise of all the talent that surged through that family. But having a child only seemed to make the marriage more incendiary and their home an inferno. The man, as often happens, was the first to bail out. He took himself off to distant Dundee on a scholarship. It was a shock for everyone. Friends lamented how beautiful they had been, how perfect together. Others were less generous.

'I have seen him talk to cacti,' said one Bong Bertie Wooster wannabe to another, in all seriousness. 'But she cries, she cries to herself all night I'm told,' offered another catty socialite. 'Can you blame her?' said someone quietly in the corner, only to be ignored.

It came as a shock to family too. Perhaps the younger sister had some inkling of the growing cracks in her sister's flawless façade, but their celebrated mother had never really looked close enough. And their doting father? Well, he thought his daughters perfect. It was hard for him to see anything beyond their brilliance. But the brilliance was brittle. In the years her husband was away, Millie's magnificent mind shattered into smithereens. Her three-year old daughter, watching from the sidelines, breathed in the dust from the wreckage.

And her father never came back. Not really. In the summer of 1955, he returned briefly to declare he would be making his home abroad. He may have even tried to persuade his wife to go with him – he certainly wanted his daughter along. But the family no longer believed the once-incandescent pair would make anything but a hash of life, so Millie's young daughter remained with her well-meaning grandparents while the father disappeared once again. And Millie? She unravelled further. Becoming reclusive, uncommunicative and then one day, just not there at all, except physically. The family, urged by friends and steered by doctors, embarked on a course of treatment that most affluent 'madwomen' (and many madmen) were subjected to at the time, in the fond belief that it would cure her.

They did the usual round of the best-known shrinks, with each offering a different solution. Some of these men suggested putting her away, but her parents were not prepared to do so. Drugs were prescribed but seemed to make no difference. Then, one day, a doctor recommended electroshock therapy. And so Millie, who had flown the coop of her 'real life' by then, was literally jolted back to earth. Except it didn't work. If anything, it may have pushed her further into the other world she inhabited.

It was done, of course, with the best possible intentions. In the 1950s, shock therapy was still very much in vogue. Introduced in 1938 and administered to millions over the next forty years, these electrically-induced seizures as a means of curing mental illness were declared 'high-risk' by the FDA in 1976 and replaced by anti-depressants. Unsurprisingly, thrice as many women as men had been subjected to ECT, even when diagnosed with the same disease. A 1974 American study found 75 per cent of ECT recommendations in Canada and 69 per cent in the US had been for women. Ernest Hemingway died after a course in 1961, but not before protesting, 'What is the sense of ruining my head and erasing my memory which is my capital, and putting me out of business? It was a brilliant cure but we lost the patient.'[18] Many other ECT patients would have said the same, but they weren't Hemingway. Most weren't even men.

ECT would go on to become one of the most reviled medical treatments in history, due in no small part to films like Ken Kesey's *One Flew Over the Cuckoo's Nest* and its depiction of shock therapy as a punishment doled out to wayward kooks. With terrible and lasting consequences. And for a long time, that was believed to be true. Recent research suggests that shock therapy is effective only half the time and never lasting in its effects, either good or bad. It also proposes that ECT has its uses and may not be the monstrous mistreatment we feared.

Sometimes seen as the only treatment in difficult circumstances like emergencies, where rapid response is required to stymie stupors, dangerous delusions or imminent suicide, it is also, allegedly, one of the few safe interventions for pregnant women (which makes me think, yay, anything to help pregnant women and then ooh, aren't these 'just-for-women' cures always dodgy?). Either way, shock therapy is back with up to one million annual subscribers in the new millennia. For Millie, however, it was an unmitigated disaster. As she slipped further away, her family went back to making desperate rounds of doctors in a last-ditch attempt to bring back their dazzling daughter. Millie carried on living – *just* – in her parents' home. Once filled with life, love and laughter, it had become a mausoleum for the living dead. The younger daughter married and moved. The fiery, famous mother passed away. Eventually the granddaughter too moved on, marrying a man who was very eligible but entirely different in temperament and ideology because, truth be told, she was in a hurry to leave that decaying lakeside house.

When Dita left, the old house lost its last bright spark and fell into a deep sleep. My great-grandfather tried to keep it going. Buying cake for his faraway-and-yet-there daughter every Friday. Rosogollas for the whole household the day after. He was a kindly man and it wasn't just sweets he handed out readily, helping the less fortunate with his money and time though he was no longer prosperous. But, like his daughter, he lived in the old house but wasn't really there anymore. His heart was now with his granddaughter and great-granddaughter halfway across the city in a long, thin pink house he travelled to nearly every day. He would arrive in his tweed suit, his walking stick by his side, and always with a satchel he kept as a memento of his elder daughter's academic exploits, in which nestled a brand new children's book and a slab of chocolate for his beloved great-granddaughter. For me.

'I've been waiting for you,' I would trill as he came through the door. 'No, don't put the book down,' he'd reply as he kissed the top of my head, settling down with his own tome and tea that had materialized at his elbow. We would read side by side, absently nibbling on cubes of chocolate. It would strike me again then how utterly happy I was for those two hours in the day when I had my 'Dadadu' beside me, though our adventures had become more and more sedentary as age and infirmity crept up on him. Isn't it lovely to be alone yet together? We don't need to be out and about or even talking, just as long as we do the things we enjoy with people who understand us, my four-year-old self would have chirped, trying to pin down an already elusive happiness in my grown-before-my-time manner.

That, while my parents worked on *their* partnership in their own if-we-don't-kill-each-other-we-would've-done-a-good-job way. 'How MUCH did you say you paid for that?' My father would say, glowering. Half my mom's monthly pay as it turned out. 'But I bought it with my own money,' she would fling back, and that was true. 'Well, you can't have it in this room,' he would insist, casting around for a reason why, his eyes alighting on the open window, 'because it will block ventilation.' At which even I, at that age, looked askance. The proposed wall for the picture was nowhere near the window and certainly not in its way.

That was the cue for my mother to take it up a notch. She would either a) cry and rue the day she married him, culminating in her tearing his new shirt, which would involve further expense, anathema to my father, or b) cry and rue the day she married him, ending with unfavourable comparisons between her family's gentility and his. He, in turn, would question the sanity of her family as a whole. All of which would take place, at least in the early days, cooped up in a small room in the long, pink house on the southern edge of the city. It was an early introduction to genetics for me. Not only did I ingest the flying dust from their discontent and make it my own, I also understood that whole families could be nuts, generation after unfortunate generation. Which turned out to be consistent with the stories that have emerged from the maternal Pandora's Box over the years; that the scourge may have extended far beyond Millie's immediate family, that it affected uncles, aunts and cousins, and their progeny to boot. A blighted bloodline, as they used to say in melodramas, but blood wasn't the problem; it was genes, instead. It has always been believed that mental illnesses, like physical ailments, can run in families. The literary Brontës, for example, were not only all predisposed to consumption but also to melancholy.

Now, of course, researchers believe there is more to it. Trauma and stress experienced in difficult situations can be passed on genetically as well. The gene itself does not alter, but the imprint left on it in the traumatized parent is passed to the child. The child is then often found to have stress disorder even if they've never had a traumatic experience themselves. That's the theory of epigenetic inheritance in the layest of layman's terms.[19] This felt like a double whammy to me: if the genes don't getcha, collateral damage from imploding parental lives will.

Dita's runaway dad, Ajit's life didn't play out the way it was meant to either. By the time my father finally caught up with his absent father-in-law, in London in the eighties, to meet the missing member of his wife's family, Ajit was a broken man, a shadow of the self who had charmed 1940s Kolkata. You might say he deserved it because he walked out on his wife and daughter, but it's never as simple as that. There doesn't have to be a villain in a family tragedy; a family can fall apart readily without one. It is a story that repeats itself over and over again around the world – the story of fragile families is the oh-so-common tale of the mismanagement of mental health problems.

It didn't stop at Millie or Ajit, the father, or even Dita. I have suffered from depression and agonizingly intense self-esteem issues all my life. And I have seen frightening signs of these in my still tenderly young son. 'Mommy, sometimes I feel sad for no reason,' he said to me one day after an unusually quiet walk home from school. I was immediately worried because that's exactly how I felt from time to time. Sad for no reason. 'Like when you do an orange poo,' he continued with the analogy most likely to strike a little boy, original thinker though he often was, 'but haven't had any orange food for days.'

I smiled and told him how I felt similarly sometimes, that it wasn't unusual, but we needed to keep talking about it. 'Talk to me when you feel sad. Maybe we can figure out what's bothering you and try to fix it.' He acquiesced and then said, 'But I wish I had a beetroot-poo mind. Bright-pink poo can only happen if you've had beetroot. Sadness should only follow something bad. Simple.' But you don't want a simple mind, my love, I thought but didn't say. I squeezed his hand instead. Like all loving parents, I want many wonderful things for both my children – health, happiness, success and intellectual accomplishments – including the complex creativity of generations of my family. But without the crazies, *please.*

Mental illnesses are no better handled now than they were in the past. Whilst sufferers are no longer seen as victims of sorcery or demonic possession by more modern societies, they are still dismissed as selfish or irresponsible, and their distress as imaginary, by the vast majority of people. But if you get the 'snap out of its' and 'pull yourself togethers' from those around you, you aren't guaranteed an easy ride from medical professionals either.

On the fringes are the quacks and their cures, from the laying of hands to swallowing fish whole. But mainstream practises can seem as experimental or misguided. Popping happy pills and getting things off your chest are advocated en masse for mental illnesses, till they acquire such alarming proportions that the heavy artillery is brought out.

This includes Transcranial Magnetic Stimulation (sending magnetic pulses through the skull), Deep Brain Treatment (inserting fine needles in the brain through small holes made in the skull), Vagus Nerve Stimulation (as vague as its name), ECT, of course, and good old-fashioned hospitalization. There are many more methods out there, some as hit and miss as the old 'cures', though more closely monitored and therefore less likely to cause death and devastation.

Yet, miscarriages of mental health justice still happen and women, inevitably, get the sharp end of the stick (or fine needle through the brain). The world insists on seeing women as less stable despite the evidence to the contrary. Serious illnesses like schizophrenia and bipolar disorder happen as often in men as women. The gender bias creeps in more often than not in their treatment. A woman is more likely to be diagnosed with depression than a man, even if they have the same symptoms. Mood-mutating drugs are also more often prescribed to women. This gender stereotyping then reinforces the age-old conditioning, which stands in the way of accurate diagnosis and proper treatment for both men and women[20].

In popular literature and films too, women have been depicted as more unbalanced. Even the most liberal of writers seem to propagate this belief. Jane Austen in *Pride and Prejudice* has Mrs Bennett suffering from 'nerves' and related imaginary ailments. But look closer, and Mr Bennett in his extreme detachment and withdrawal from home and hearth is equally unbalanced. And who's to say that 'mad' Mrs Rochester in Jane Eyre didn't flip her lid *after* her marriage to a most peculiar man? In the real world, history heaves with stories of mad women. But that's because it's always been convenient to regard women as crazy if they flouted the social strictures that unfairly bound them. The easiest way to discredit and even dispose of such women was to question their sanity. This was a tack taken by some very canny men fairly early, and the method stuck because it worked, and the more it worked the more people used this as a weapon against women who were in their way. So even more women were recorded as mad, giving the myth of feminine imbalance further credence.

Tina Fey said, 'The definition of crazy in show business is a woman who keeps talking after no one wants to fuck her anymore[21].' In other words, a woman becomes 'crazy' when she's no longer nubile or acquiescent, and has started stating inconvenient truths to boot. She's also a threat if she scandalously tries to take control of her property and/or sexuality.

Clip the Clit!

Hysteria was also conveniently seen as a feminine affliction, caused by 'sex-starved' or roving wombs. Of this, Plato said very wisely (as Plato always did, even when he had no clue – a special talent possessed by Leaders of Men): 'If the uterus remains unfruitful long beyond its proper time, it gets discontented and angry and wanders in every direction through the body, closing up the passages of breath, and, by obstructing respiration, drives women to extremity.'

Doctors through the ages, therefore, worked away busily at soothing the womb, arriving at methods that ranged from the mild to the malevolent. From forcing women to inhale fumes from things reeking or rank to repel the womb from the respiratory tract, to hectoring them into marriage and childbirth (wombs always returned to their rightful place for baby-bearing, after all), they inflicted every kind of horror on their patients in the name of treatment.[22] In Victorian times, for example, women displaying signs of excitability even under the most extreme pressure were frequently clapped into asylums for their hysteria; they were also put in the care of doctors who often colluded in dispossessing or disinheriting them.

But when it came to misguided or malicious cures, the clitoridectomy beat them all hands down (conceived, ironically, to deter women from doing precisely that). Clits – sensory locus of a woman's lust, and her wings, were clipped alike to prevent her from straying or *worse*, pleasuring herself (both, symptoms of hysteria as well, apparently). The haste to inflict this on women died down in the West in the late 1800s, though in Africa, it continues to be forced upon millions of women. However, hysteria as a feminine malady lasted another century. Yet if women today are spared at least that, they continue to be viewed as madder than men. Especially at 'that time of the month'.

The Hulk in a Pretty Frock

Remember snip-snipping Lorena Bobbitt? Apparently, she was menstruating. And who doesn't know that menstruating women are terribly, horribly mad? And dangerous. But this is untrue, and we are not flakey and unreliable for seven days out of a month. It's not as if we'd be let off with murder if we committed it while menstruating. Noooo, *that* degree of mad would be unacceptable. It should be just enough to allow men to make light of our skills and credibility and elbow us out of desirable situations, and no more.

And those stories we've all heard about women running amuck whilst bleeding? They are down to extreme provocation, plain old criminal intent or some other form of mental illness altogether. I say 'other', but premenstrual syndrome or PMS is not an illness at all; it is a perfectly normal physiological condition affecting at least 85 per cent of all women. Men have hormonal surges too. Pulitzer Prize-winning writer Maureen Dowd finds these stereotypical signs of PMS just as common in men, 'Women are affected by lunar tides only once a month but men have raging hormones every day, as we noticed when Dick Cheney rampaged around the globe like Godzilla[23].' We all know Godzilla-like men. Think ISIS if you aren't convinced.

On the other hand, PMS, in its most severe form, known as PMDD or Premenstrual Dysphoric Disorder, affects only 3 per cent of women and seldom leads to violence. I can get awfully blue at that time of the month. I might shout more than usual but I'm rarely moved to murder! But if I am, it will have more to do with all the rottenness in the world than my menstrual cycle.

Post-partum's No Party

Post-partum depression isn't much fun either. It sounds simple: a dramatic drop in hormones like estrogen and progesterone causes it, often in combination with other bodily imbalances. It affects up to a quarter of all new mothers, but could happen just as well to the mother-who-never-got-to-be. The symptoms, however, are far from simple, ranging from mild irritability that disappears in a fortnight to hallucinations and self-harming tendencies that can dog a woman for years. Consolation is often offered to these women with sops both trite and flowery, and completely inadequate.

No matter how you dress it, you can't make either post-partum depression or a miscarriage pretty or heart-warming. It doesn't feel like a wiped-clean, daisy-scented fresh start you can embark on because Baby's definitely gone. No, it feels like a nasty spreading stain that takes over your whole life. What is even more devastating is when you're hit by post-partum depression after a miscarriage. That's a low blow indeed.

It takes various shapes in various women. In me, it manifested itself as hopelessness, loneliness and self-hate, needing endless validation. Eager (for) beavers with anything but good intentions came forward in droves to tell me how wonderful I was. And I wanted to hear it. I needed to hear it to keep me going from day to day.

So, when an erudite and entertaining senior civil servant f(r)iend, who usually discussed Osaka and Ogden Nash online, insisted, 'Send me a picture of your ass,' I sidestepped with a mock-vapid, 'but I don't own a donkey.' But he wasn't about to let it go. 'A picture of your ripe, rounded, scrumptious double-plum rump.' 'Bottom selfies are impossible to take,' I said struggling to stay good-humoured. 'In a gimp suit then,' he instructed, 'pour yourself into one. You have one don't you, adventurous lady that you are? Your heaving bosom (he was of a certain age) straining against leather, with a whip in your hand. Something I can take to the Governor's ante-room for my afternoon indulgence.' It was the first I'd heard of his activities in the afternoon, and I SO did not indulge him.

Far too many such virtual friends would start off suave and sensitive, and end up seedy. To begin with, they loved my writing, commended my mothering and serenaded my smile, and that would keep me buoyed for a while, but then almost inevitably, it would turn ugly. And I would feel dirty from their blandishments, though from so far away. Or unworthy of attention as they moved on to more accommodating souls online.

My need for such insincere solace (though I almost never saw that it was insincere till it was too late) was sending me spiralling further into the abyss. But turning elsewhere, I would be beset with the regulatory exhortations to 'snap out of it', 'get over it', and 'move on with your life'. I also got 'it was never even a baby'. All very well-meaning, I'll grant you, yes, even that last remark, but it left me not just astounded but sadder still. Couldn't they tell I was trying precisely to get over it, snap out of it? Couldn't they see the malevolent gooey mess that was holding me in place as I struggled and failed to get free? Like Ricky Gervais, I should have said, 'Telling people with depression to snap out of it is about as useful as telling people with cancer to stop having cancer[24].'

But I didn't know until months later that it was postpartum depression, that my hormones were causing havoc. Had I known, could I have dealt with it better? Maybe. I did do something that might have been the saving of me. This, and my husband's steadfast support, regardless of what I threw at him, saw me through the stickiest patch. I decided to put some distance between myself and the drama that had played itself out in my beautiful home in Sherwood Forest. Picturesque though it was, I needed a fresh start in a place that had walls and trees and an expanse of sky that looked significantly different, but was familiar and comfortable at the same time. A fresh start in an old sanctuary.

So, I took myself and my two little ones back to the city of my birth. This was the only place on earth where the smell of day-old puddles, nose-prickling mustard oil and the smoky scent of a quick-falling dusk combine to create a comforting aroma. It was time to allow myself to be gathered back into the womb of the strangely tall and narrow house I grew up in. It was time to give myself the latitude to let go: of Baby, online attachments and all the tumult of that summer. And the place to do it in was a rosy room in a pink house with books stacked to the ceiling and an unobstructed view over the tops of coconut trees all the way to the tracks in the distance.

It was time to return to Kolkata.

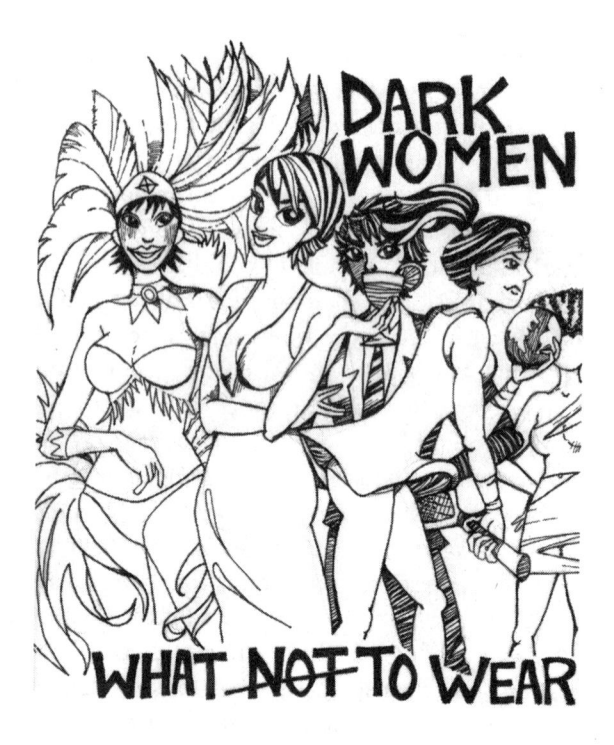

6

You Taste of Chocolate, Girl

In what was then the southern edge of Kolkata, a little girl was born in the seventies. She almost arrived in her house rather than the fancy hospital arranged for the purpose because Kolkata was under water that late-August morning. But her father was young and intrepid (*and* worried about having to deliver the child himself), so he ensured his sturdy little car ploughed through walls of water to get his wife and his almost-there daughter to the hospital in time. This little girl, not being content with just lying there, as any good baby would, had been exploring the dark world of the womb and, having felt the need to turn round and round again in her search for answers, had wound the umbilical cord around herself several times.

It would have been quite harmless if the umbilical cord had coiled around her waist but, as with everything she did, here too, she caused the worst possible result: the cord tightened itself round her neck. She was therefore the result of an emergency caesarean. But mother and child were happy and healthy and hyperactive (more child than mother) within hours of the delivery. What she was not (the baby, that is, because the mother certainly was and had the name Tuktuki or Rosy to show for it) was light-skinned. And this became one of the most noted things about the bright-eyed baby over the next few days. So much so that someone dared ask the celebrated great-grandmother whether she thought the baby's skin colour was a disappointment, considering the pale tones of the mom.

The fiery eighty-year-old fixed the quailing visitor with an obelisk-like glare, and said, 'Colour? The colour of her skin? What I see is a girl who will go far!' The criticism of my darker skin had drawn her ire, and I had got myself a character certificate in my first two days of life from one of Bengal's premier women novelists. She died soon after though, and outside my family, her spirited exhortation to see past my skin tone never cut any ice.

Besides the bigger, utterly infuriating issue of lighter skin being accepted as better, without rhyme, reason or demur, there's the quibbling over minute differences in shade that makes it murkier still (see, see, it's entrenched in language even). It's impossible not to cotton on early that in half the world, and certainly in India, you are seen as inferior because you are a micro-shade darker than someone else. Often, the difference is so small that people of another race, notably Caucasians, our yardstick in all this, can't even spot it.

Two sisters I knew were strikingly different shades of brown. Everybody felt the need to comment on it. One of the sisters – the fairer one, as it so happened – married a European man. At her wedding reception, the Old Wives huddled around for their usual game of snide and hurtful compare-the-sisters'-skin-tones. Always within earshot of the darker one. This time though, they were also trying to impress the European contingent sitting close by. So they spoke in loud stage whispers, hoping to draw the latter into the conversation about the two sisters' looks.

'Look at Shona, so bright, so goldy, marrying your rosy boy, no? But Nina, what to do with Nina? She is so dull in colour that she could only get a Bengali boy,' said an aunty wreathed in smiles. 'So ugly she is,' added the anorexic young lady in a blinding lehenga sitting beside the aunties, hoping to score *brownie* points with the gora log. 'But what to do,' another aunty carped, 'such a black-black colour can be ugly only.'

The gora log, in the meantime, were looking bemused. Finally, the groom's brother, no less, piped up with a look of utter surprise on his face, 'But aren't Nina and Shona the same colour?' The horror on the aunties' faces had to be seen to be believed. They could not understand it. The knowledge of what was or wasn't beautiful had formed the bedrock of all their beliefs and here it had been neatly dismantled in a single sentence. For a whole six months after, they steered clear of sniping at Nina for the 'dirtiness' of her skin.

But Nina was not alone. Most dark-skinned Indian women, and even men of a dusky persuasion, have had to put up with hurtful words, a narrower band of opportunities and sometimes (though fortunately, rarely) sticks and stones. Here, for your entertainment (of course it is, haven't you noticed how Bollywood buffoons are mostly dark too?) are some popular forms of dark-skin baiting.

1. 'How can you play Sita when you're so black?' Or just swop that name for any central character in Indian literature and that's what most of us would have heard growing up. School plays are a staple of any child's existence and getting a stellar role depends on everything but your ability to act. In the West, the nativity is the thing to be in, and whether you are cast as Second Lobster (you didn't know about the lobsters in the manger?) or Angel Gabriel tells you a *fair* bit about what the teachers think of you, but less and less does it have to do with skin colour. After all, my beautiful cappuccino-coloured five-year-old daughter played Mother Mary, at the heart of the Nativity, last Christmas. As Mary is viewed as indubitably white by all self-respecting English people, giving this role to a non-white child would have been unthinkable a decade ago.

    In India though, this fine tradition continues and children are excluded from pivotal parts in school performances, sports and even academic opportunities if they don't look 'bright' enough. But 'bright' in India rarely means clever, oh no, 'bright' means fair-skinned. And children, vulnerable and impressionable, often get overlooked because they are too dark. Odiousness rating 9 (on a scale of 1 to 10).

2. And let's not even go into the lexicon of colour hang-

ups. Actually, shall we? It's time we turned the tables and laughed at *them*. Amongst the many wonderful things you get called in Bengal alone for being dark is 'moila' (dirty), 'blackie' (who doesn't love imported abuse?), or the more rustic 'keltu'. When they're trying to be kind, they might call you 'ujjwal shyamborno', the strangely oxymoronic (not to mention moronic) 'bright-dark' skin, as if a distinction has to be made because your average, everyday dark skin is always dull and murky. Anyone with eyes can see there's more sheen to mahogany than to larch.

But, blinded by prejudice, so many can't see the obvious. And if they ever feel cornered into admitting a dark person may be half-decent to look at, wait for the BUT. 'You are dark BUT attractive,' they will say, as if you couldn't be dark AND attractive. And forget beautiful. Nobody would ever call a dark person beautiful, not in most of Asia. Because they can't be, right? Since it has everything to do with the shade of skin and nothing to do with pleasing features, great hair, a dazzling smile and a body that turns up the heat. So, take that, Nandita Das! Know your place! The Rakhi Sawants are so much more than you. Odiousness rating: 7

3. Reserved for dark women is a special kind of concern. It starts with what you can and cannot wear, and finishes with how to behave. Because dark women need to be extra-demure, extra-virtuous and extra-obedient to nab a husband, any husband at all. But first, you cannot wear black, it will simply merge with your skin and people might think you're naked, tsk, tsk (and that's a death knell for your marriage

chances, Chocolate Girl). Well, guess what, mausi? Nothing suits me quite so well as an LBD, and a tiny one to boot, to show off as much of my mocha skin as possible. In black and nearly naked, all at the same time – gasp! You shouldn't wear gold either. Gold is for the 'goldy-skinned', a mausi standard meaning 'light'. In fact, dark women shouldn't wear anything that attracts attention. That's *plain* crass. As I said earlier, know your place, dark women. It is ten steps behind your lighter counterparts, where lesser people should be. Odiousness rating: 8

4. You get propositioned, not proposed to. First they convince you you're unattractive. Grinding your self-esteem to the ground, they make you feel unworthy of their attention. Having done that, they move in for the kill. You are by then too depressed to wonder why they want to nail you. No, not the mausis. Their sons. Why do they want to do you when they think it's infradig to woo you? They can't help it though, poor sods, their instincts draw them to you, as much as to any gora girl. So, what do they do? They try to have their ladoos and eat them too; wheedling the dusky one into bed before taking the pasty one home to Mommy. Odiousness rating: 6 (because you can't help but enjoy their confusion).

5. And then there's the difficult, nay, nearly impossible task of getting a dark girl married off. We all hold our breath then and await the MATRIMONIAL AD. It will have to sing our praises, yes, even us dark women. How to do that when we have nothing to recommend us? And to complicate matters, the ad needs to have a modicum of truth so the prospective groom and his

family don't walk out at first sight. A tricky one, but the coven's more than equal to it. They have come up with codes that convey to the man's family that the woman they are offering up for marriage is dark, yes, but she's not super-dark like a rakshasa; instead, she is 'wheatish'. Or she may be dark but look, look, she's tall and also a doctor. It doesn't end there. If the dark woman manages to find a mausi-sanctioned man who can overlook her colouring (because, of course, you can find unconventional, open-minded men who do, but they won't be mausi-approved, will they), then she's on her way to the next round of ritual matrimonial humiliation. First, there's the bridal makeup, a headache to one and all when the bride is dusky. She has to be made to look halfway decent somehow. That can only mean tons of talcum powder to the rescue! Slathered all over the poor woman's face and neck, its ghostly (should that be ghastly?) layers will neither match any other part of her body, nor stay on under the hot lights, peeling off in the most unattractive manner (but that's to be expected, moan the mausis, dark brides *are* unattractive – what to do). Sigh. That's me sighing this time, not the mausis. Odiousness rating: 8

6. I was going to *Dove*tail my thoughts on dark-bride dowry with the point above, but really, it deserves an outing on its own. Yes, it's that special. We all know dowry is still demanded (and given), although not always overtly. Whichever way it happens, the groom's relatives can be expected to extract their collective weight in costly stuff from the bride's family, because they are in a position of power. When the bride is

dusky, the groom's family feels even more entitled and further demands start rolling in.

Till the latter are well and truly rolling in it! The rise in dowry demands in India (there's one dowry death every hour now, up 20 per cent in the last decade), means families of brides are under more pressure than ever. Can you imagine how bad it is, therefore, for the dark-skinned girl and her family? I know of a dark girl from an underprivileged home whose single mother (practically single since her husband was always slumped over, drunk) felt compelled to marry her off to the first fella who said 'aye'. But she'd extracted that aye artfully, with layers of lightening makeup on her dusky daughter placed in a strategically lit room.

The chap's parents smelt a rat, however, and sprung a surprise visit on them, and the girls' Achilles heel was revealed. The chastisement that followed only made the girl's family feel doubly beholden. The boy's side were doing them a favour anyway, but now, they would do it despite the deceit. Naturally, their big heart went hand in hand with a large appetite: for expensive gadgets, fancy gizmos and gold ornaments too. For all of which the girl's mother had to beg or borrow, leaving her with little more than the clothes on her broken back. Odiousness rating: 10, and then some!

7. Did I mention the skin-scouring darker women are subjected to from an early age? They've trowelled it all on, from stinging lemon juice and scratchy papaya peel that cosmetic 'experts' swear by ('Rub papaya pulp on tanned skin as it is a natural skin-lightening agent,' lectures the *Times of India*), to the seriously harmful bleaches being advertized and sold.

Amongst skin specialists, 16 per cent warn against the application of such creams, while 80 per cent suggest that only those prescribed should be used. This is hardly surprising, since these lotions are almost always lethal potions of steroids, hydroquinone, and tretinoin. Over time, they can leave skin burnt, parchment-thin or ravaged by conditions like ochronosis, a hyper-pigmentation that turns skin dark purple. These creams can also be behind liver damage, mercury poisoning and The Big C – not only skin cancer but blood cancers like leukaemia and those of the liver and kidneys (can I have that papaya peel back, please).

And if the harm it does to your skin and your health wasn't bad enough, it decimates your self-confidence. How does a young woman feel, d'ya think, when she's told from day one that she's flawed, even inferior, and must do everything possible – things injurious or worse – to improve herself? She needs improvement so bad that she must put her life on the line. How would that make her feel about herself? How would it affect everything else in her life? You get the picture. None of it is *fair* or *lovely*. Actually it is, but only for the manufacturers who make millions from our ingrained self-loathing. And for the Bollywood superstars who avariciously and irresponsibly flog these products.

There are a hundred such nasty swills swanning about acting the saviour and doing our youngsters incalculable harm. But we don't care, or there wouldn't be popular spin-offs in this hideous, self-flagellating business of skin-whitening. The most famous of these festering face creams, for example, also offers a Facebook app with which we can lighten the skin-tone in our pictures. This appalling app is plugged pertly by pale-from-birth pretty boy Shahid Kapur. The boy wants to go global, so what better vehicle than the massive, money-spinning $10 billion skin-lightening industry? Not to be left behind, Kareena Kapoor did her bit for Blanchers Inc. when she labelled the much hotter, determinedly dusky Bipasha Basu a 'kali billi'. Worth a cheer though that Bips' rejoinder put the boot in for the dark side: 'It's bizarre, this obsession with fair skin. It reflects a lack of intelligence; something is wrong with their heads.'

It's a wonder there's anyone in Bollywood speaking up for the dark-skinned because dusky actresses can be counted on the fingers of one hand. And I mean all the way from inception to modern times. The aforementioned Nandita is another dark beauty who speaks her mind: 'We keep saying things like "uska rang saaf hai", as if dark skin is a dirty thing. This mindset is then propagated in our songs, stories and movies.'

Bollywood Queen, Kangana Ranaut, turned down a very lucrative fairness cream endorsement campaign. The incandescent King Khan, on the other hand, does yeoman service for the bleaching industry, though some of us can remember when he was a not-nearly-as-luminescent fauji in the eighties. Can you really expect Hari, Pari and Manjari to resist the promise of glow-in-the-dark skin when its champions are to be found amongst the country's great and good?

It's such an unequal battle in a nation where even children are fair game. As much as 13 per cent of the skin-whitening market is made up of twelve to fourteen-year olds! And why not? After all, isn't it the Indian way? Like cricket or Bollywood, this aspiration to be lily-white is *who we are*, based as it is on 'varna' or colour, like Hinduism itself. Odiousness rating: waaaay over 10.

A colonial hangover, however, does appear to be a pan-Asian rather than just an Indian thing. Colour discrimination is a way of life in most Asian countries. While the vaginal whitening cream first made its mark (where the sun don't shine) in India, it spread like VD to countries like Thailand. Their ad featured a disembodied voice (God?) reassuring a pale Thai girl in tight shorts which had discoloured her skin, that the vaginal whitening cream would turn her nether regions to 'bright and translucent' once again.[25] Feel right at home, don't you?

I experienced it personally in the Philippines where, for five years between six and eleven, I was constantly reminded my dark skin was 'pangit' (ugly). I can recall one Christmas with friends of my family where people kept walking up to us to give my much-paler sister brightly wrapped gifts. I waited my turn with an excited smile of anticipation, being only seven, till the umpteenth person walked away without a second glance at me. I finally realized that the 'pangit' do not receive presents.

I drowned my sorrows in delicious honey-glazed ham after. Overindulging to such an extent, I chucked it up on one of the people who hadn't thought it worthwhile to get me a gift (they got a return gift though, didn't they?). Most of all, I have ensured my children will never go through that. As the mother of one light-skinned and one darker child, I make absolutely sure no one, no matter who they are, how elderly, or how revered, dares to compare their skin tones, or lavish attention on one but not the other for their colour.

And we call it a colonial hangover. If we're honest though, we'll have to admit that colour discrimination was practised habitually and aggressively in India, and perhaps most of Asia, long before the firangis arrived, although their presence undoubtedly made things much worse. They institutionalized the practise, as we know, with jobs, schooling and other social and economic opportunities becoming the preserve of the pale-skinned. Even murder was no longer murder if the man killed was dark.

In modern times, the poster boy for colour discrimination has got to be the US, leaving South Africa far behind! With hundreds of years of slavery behind it, and a disproportionate number of black Death Row inmates currently (42 per cent, when the black population in the US is only 13.6 per cent of the whole)[26], the US is powering ahead after Donald Trump's election to the presidency, with a rising tide of discrimination and racially-motivated violence against its non-white denizens. In early 2017, two Indian men, Alok Madasani and Srinivas Kuchibhotla, working as engineers in Kansas were shot while drinking quietly in a sports bar when a white man opened fire on them, shouting 'Immigrants go home'. In the UK, a third of those shot by the police since 2004 are believed to be from black and ethnic minority communities which make up only 8 per cent of the total population.

And yet. Yet, bizarrely, in social situations, I have faced far less racism in England, my second home, than I have in India. Even as we hate the white man for the pernicious practice of racism, when it comes to picking a life partner, they seem to choose on the basis of skin colour less often. At least not the liberal, educated classes, though the same cannot be said of their Indian counterparts. Of the Caucasian and Asian men I have dated, the former have proudly introduced me to their parents, while the latter have struggled with bringing me home to their mommies. It baffled me till an epidermal twin spelt it out in black and white, 'We are well-educated, well-dressed, well-spoken and well-behaved; there can be no other reason but our skin colour.'

One experience in particular, involving an Indian man who actually shoved me into a putrid cupboard when his mother turned up, brought it home to me. Minutes before, he had been holding my hand, looking into my eyes and telling me he loved me, swearing he wanted to live his life with me, and that marriage was the only answer to the life-long longing he knew he would feel for me (it was so corny I should've known, but I *was* nineteen). His other hand had found its way to my bra clasp and undone it, but since I didn't consider love and sex mutually exclusive in that Indo-Victorian way, I found no cause for alarm there.

His mouth clamped down on mine, pumping hot air into me (he certainly had an excess of it; was he trying to give some away?). His fingers, in the meantime, had snaked into my sensible white cotton bra, grasping and squeezing my breast as if he were testing fruit for ripeness. It must have passed muster as he swooped down the very next moment, intending to wrap his tongue around it. But then his head jerked back violently, as if an invisible leash had been pulled. And that's just what it was. His mother was unexpectedly at the front door.

'Beta, there is a double lock on. Has Ramu done that? Will that idiot never learn! Come and open up for me, sweetie.' The next thing I know, I'm being shoved into a large closet full of shoes and shawls, reeking of sweat and guilt. Not mine but his. Naturally, that relationship didn't come to fruition! Not so much for my time in his cupboard as for his admission weeks later that he could never have introduced me to Mommy. *She* wanted someone pale and traditional.

Though never quite so dramatically again, the Indian male reluctance to bring dusky women home to their mothers continued to be a part of my life, though mostly experienced vicariously thereafter as I turned my attentions elsewhere. That's not to say I didn't meet any nice Indian boys. Like the sweet, shorn Sikh boy who put me on a pedestal, introduced me to his truly lovely mother, encouraging us to become friends, and we did. But my friendship with *him* floundered as he turned out to be too nice for an adventurous girl like me.

Is my life colour-discrimination free now? Hell, no. I've faced it in England while seeking employment 'beyond my station' as a brown-skinned immigrant woman who is clearly meant to stay home and cook curries. Or at best, work at a call centre. Which happens to be the first job I did get in the UK (but this woman doesn't cook curries; she cooks up plans and then follows them through till she's back doing what she does best). I've faced discrimination trying to buy ice cream at an evil little shop in a forgotten corner of Cornwall. And I've had to, with my heart breaking, live it through my children when they've come home with stories of indignities suffered in the playground, though these occurrences have been rare compared to my experiences in India and the Philippines.

There is no perfect place. But if you weigh up the insults I have endured in England against twenty years' worth in India, and the abuse all dark-skinned Indians put up with daily, the colour of your skin will scar you far worse in the Motherland than almost anywhere else. So you flee your outrageously complexion-constricted life to freedom, choice and appreciation in a foreign clime. There, you are not 'kalo' or 'moila' anymore. You are deliciously dusky, scrumptiously chocolatey and terrifically tanned. Best of all, you and your lovely, equally dusky daughter will never have to look upon a tube of skin-whitening cream for as long as you both shall live.

7

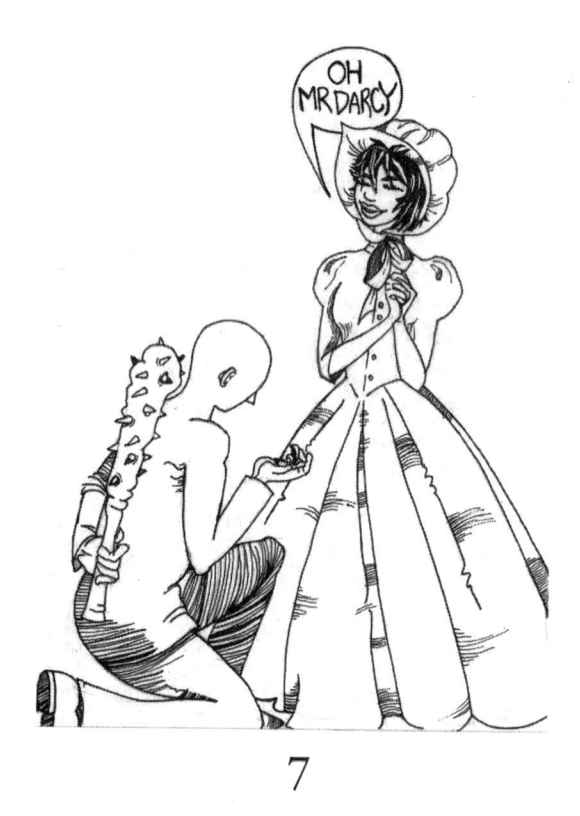

Hit Me Baby One More Time

Sherwood Forest is beautiful at any time of the year. In the summer, it's a rich golden-green, full of bird song and adventure. But in the winter, when it's stark, dark and scary, it's no less stunning. Leached of life and colour, it takes on an air of mystery. In our roomy red-brick home, that's just grist for the mill. It's a backdrop on which we pin our numerous fantastical but deeply pleasing stories!

'Did you spot him, Mommy?' Anika breathed, her button nose pasted to the kitchen pane. Out in the gloaming, the trees whispered conspiratorially as the shadows shifted to form a large apelike creature, shuffling noisily towards us. She dashed to the wide glass garden doors, feverishly working the handle, 'It's Critterpitapatus! He's coming this way!' I ran to help her lock it in case they were frightened. 'Oh Mommy,' she said, 'geddaway!' And she flung the doors wide open joyfully.

Critterpitapatus shambled in with a grunt and a heave. Then Daddy put the large dun sack of weatherproofs and wellies down on our grooved wooden floor with a thud. 'All set for our forest trek, kids!' he grin-puffed, apelike and shambling no more. The next day, after our ramble, we wrote our second Critterpitapatus story, with hoots of laughter and some stealthy ink-slinging.

It's not just food for thought this forest gives us, but the stuff of life too: trees laden with fruit, mushrooms underfoot, lush little glades for sanctuary on difficult days … nearly everything I could have asked for. Here, our days and nights are busy, happy and fulfilling. Of course, there are trials, tribulations and tantrums too: the grazed knees and tomato-thieving squirrels; mock-serious spats on the appropriate time for bed and the husband's mislaid keys!

But did such bliss happen in the blink of an eye? With the wave of a magic wand the minute I moved to England? Did it all fall into place like a fairy story? Far from it. The road from south Kolkata to Sherwood Forest turned out to be long, hard and rocky. I nearly didn't find it at all. I even took an unlikely detour via Sheffield and almost lost my way, no, not *in* the woods, but on the way there. It was the woods, after all, that I needed to reach before I could tell my story. Because this is a story that requires several deep gulps of pure Sherwood air. A cuddle from my kids and a steaming cup of cocoa. For courage.

Oh Mr Darcy!

You'd think I'd have learnt my lesson after my experience with Duncan, wouldn't you? But the more I knew of Indian men, the less they seemed likely to work for me. And the more I sought escape in English novels and Hollywood movies, the more my body and brain (and heart!) craved a dashing storybook hero, romantic and rugged at the same time.

Yet, I should have remembered to be careful with what I wished for, because one walked into my life soon after. An Englishman called George, what else? Blue-eyed and romantic, yes, but neither dashing nor heroic, and sadly devoid of chin. The fact that he didn't seem particularly polished or bright I chose to overlook as superficial; his heart seemed in the right place (so what was a missing brain?). Most of all, he was devoted. It was usually me who got in too deep, and got hurt. Instead, here was a man who appeared willing to move heaven and earth to keep me by him. He was attached in a way no one had been before. And I wasn't wrong about that. Just about everything else.

Besides, at twenty-five, I had grown distinctly broody. Bridget Jones broody, and with just as little sense when it came to matters of the heart. So I found myself visiting him in wind-blown Sheffield in northern England. On our way there in his great, big roaring beast of a car – a Jaguar – we drove through elegant cities, picturesque towns and the quaintest of villages.

There was so much to see and get to know of this gorgeous new country, that I wasn't sizing up my new man like a clever girl should. He seemed a nice, steady, dependable sort of fellow – what more could there be to him, I thought. And that was enough for a holiday romance, wasn't it? It was never meant to be more than that, and I approached it as such, feeling carefree, hedonistic and even frivolous.

Trouble was that in front of grand Chatsworth in the rolling Derbyshire Dales, the estate on which Jane Austen had based Darcy's magnificent Pemberley, he got down on one knee and popped the question. And I found myself saying yes. That it felt unreal seemed right somehow, since I'd grown up with the belief that that's what romance was meant to be – woozy, like the feeling that I am overcome by before one of my epileptic fits, though more pleasant, one hoped, than the fit itself. Except that our marriage worked out to be exactly like one of my epileptic fits, dreamy in the run up, and bruising after.

Just before my English holiday, work for Rupert Murdoch had become exceptionally unexciting. Therefore, boredom, a sense of hopelessness with romances never quite working out, a need for adventure and my new lover's twinkling eyes (which later seemed pebble-hard and baleful) led me to marry thoughtlessly. I became an accidental settler in Sheffield, leaving behind everything I knew, everything that made me who I was – my urbane family and friends, successful career and relatively sophisticated pursuits ... in fact, my whole identity and with it, my self-esteem. Yet, I thought all this a fair swap for a shiny new adventure in a brand new place.

Yuletide Surprise

My exciting adventure, however, died young. Our romance lasted as long as we toured England with our Jaguar ('ours' as I was encouraged to believe; later revealed to be hired) purring through banks of hedgerow, down narrow country lanes, under yew tree and oak, with birds chirruping on every branch. The greenness of the landscape, the creaminess of the clotted cream that crowned our wayside scones and the glow cast by this little island's long list of literary lights, whose legacy was simply everywhere, from lovingly preserved historic buildings to many-storeyed bookstores, everything I fell in love with while exploring England died a death once we settled in Sheffield.

The city, at the turn of the century, was moribund with that moss-damp smell and underfoot-squelch of a cemetery after the rains. With the same graveyard stillness. I woke to a town trapped in a time warp, still mourning its destruction in World War II and the demise of its steel industry. Every bit the city of *The Full Monty* but with a thick black vein of deep despair I was unprepared for. It was green but forever obscured by grey sheets of rain. The clotted cream was no less creamy but with a bitter aftertaste as my marriage went sour. And violent as my new husband turned out to have the pugilistic predilections of every disaffected man in the gritty, low-cost northern English films I'd seen. And he didn't even look like Sean Bean!

As our marriage went belly-up, I blamed myself for it (as we women have always been told to). I blamed myself for having wedded chalk to cheese, which is what we were. We were from vastly different backgrounds. Class, education, values and personalities – none of it matched. What had seemed exotic and therefore exciting, now felt plain wrong. But I had worked myself into a state of love for him and found it difficult to walk away.

He had changed from someone who promised to look after me (and yes, I shouldn't need that but I think I had always wanted a port in a storm more than anything else) to a man-child who needed looking after constantly. He had seemed sensible, practical and financially comfortable, but turned out to be in shitloads of debt. I thought his dependable, solid nature would make him an excellent father when the time came, but I was wrong there too. Solid soon turned out to be stolid and worse. He was not the calm, quiet individual I thought him to be, as I discovered on our first Christmas together, two months after we got married.

My first Christmas in England was meant to be magical. I had wonderful memories of the Yuletide season in Catholic Philippines. Once again, I had that breathless feeling leading up to the holidays. I had a tree to put up, baubles to festoon it with, festive food to work my way through and gifts to buy and receive, with all the excitement of a seven-year-old once more. I meticulously set the stage for the most romantic Christmas ever. My new husband seemed equally excited and happily did his bit, getting tangled in the Christmas lights and sharpening carving knives for the planned traditional dinner.

I didn't know though that the knives were out for *me*. I cannot now remember what had triggered it, but one minute we were talking merrily about dinner and the next, he was coming at me with fists swinging. It was the first time and I couldn't believe it was happening. So, I froze like a rabbit caught in the headlights but when it looked like he would really hit me, that it wasn't some strange Yorkshire yuletide surprise, I made a run for it but up the stairs to the attic room instead of out of the house. He caught up with me as I was trying to shut the door on him and his fist connected with my left eye. I still remember what that felt like because it was a first. Blazing pain mixed with a cold horror. I heard the clock ticking on our landing as I waited for something else to happen, even just my response. I had no clue what that should be. As screechy, screamy and turbulent as my parents' marriage was, we were gentle folk, and the very idea of fisticuffs was abhorrent.

But when I didn't react, he did. He dissolved into tears. He hadn't meant for that to happen. He had lost it. He was abandoned at the age of two by a heartless mother. And what I'd said had reminded him of her (what had I said? His fist had wiped it from my memory). But he loved me really. 'Will it ever happen again?' I questioned coolly, considering the turmoil inside and the throbbing mass that was my face. He promised it never would. But looking back now, I realize there was a caveat I had failed to spot. It would never happen again *if* I did as told. It was my fault that Christmas and my fault every time it happened thereafter. And the responsibility for covering up for him – lying to my parents, editing photographs with tell-tale signs, was also mine.

A Tale as Old as Time

I know this is a *strikingly* familiar story for abused women everywhere. So many women have been through this arc with their intimate abusers. First, there is the complete absence of such tendencies. Then, perhaps only a hint of something. Maybe possessiveness. George used to like telling me he would chop off my head if I ever looked at another man. To someone like me, weaned on romantic fiction, that just sounded like an OTT protestation of love. And you don't take it seriously of course, not to start with.

Then it worsens. Threats begin to get carried out. 'Did you like Tom, my old friend,' he might say very innocently about a man he'd introduced me to that day. 'Such a nice man,' I might gush to make him happy, not mentioning Tom's bad breath or wandering eye. Something catches *my* eye even as I say this. It's his fist, it's coming at me and it's too late to duck. On occasion, it's not his fist but his fingers tightening round my neck or a foot swinging into my ribs once I'm down. Sometimes feet (if like me, you are waiflike) kick you clear off the stairs, leaving you lying dazed and bruised at the bottom.

Then you lie there not making a sound. Not only because it's the easiest way to end the episode *and* defeat him (he wants to hear your pain, after all), but also because you're too stunned to react. Once again. In fact, that's how you stay for a good few years. As it worsens and takes new turns, the full horror of your situation is revealed to you, but you are still in denial. Because right after he's hit you, the mind games start and no amount of smarts on your part helps you cope with the cunning manipulations of a man you've grown attached to. The tears (his!), the turning of the tables, the promises to behave with a corollary, always, that implies the woman is the responsible party. She made him hurt her. She needs to toe his line, *she* needs to sort herself out.

And why did I fall for it? Because I was psychologically battered, shocked, hurt and disillusioned, a weakened version of who I used to be. I, like countless other women, wanted to cling to the hope that things could not be as bad as they seemed. Someone we decided to love couldn't be so terrible, could they? Could they? How did we get it so wrong?

Sounds nuts, doesn't it? Yet there are so many of us, way more than you think, because so few admit to their 'shame'. Only 10 per cent, it is believed, come forward. And it's never the perpetrator who's laid low by the thought of what he's done; it's always us women. I say 'women' knowingly, because although men can be victims of domestic violence, more than 80 per cent of such abuse worldwide, especially of an intimate or severe nature, happens to women.

You might think that your own husband beating you up is Neanderthal, and has got to be on the wane, right? On the contrary, a 2013 report showed an 11 per cent rise in domestic violence in Britain, 70 per cent in Australia over three years, and a mind-boggling 134 per cent in the last ten years in India.

Even if the jump can be explained merely by the fact that more women are reporting such crimes, the figures still astound.

And this has nothing to do with being weak. Abused women are *not* doormats. So many bright, vibrant, successful, even strong, women fall into this trap. I'd like to believe I was one too, if very immature and confused by the strangeness of the situation. And how about the celebrities? How about Nigella Lawson? Domestic Goddess, Old Money, beautiful and successful – who would dare mess with her? Her husband, Charles Saatchi, that's who. Not so long ago, she was plastered across every paper with her face white with shock and her husband gripping her by the throat. Yup, Britain has just woken up to the fact that their upper classes get battered too, with a significant rise in domestic crimes against professional women reported in recent years.

There are so many other celebrity cases one can mention. Ike's leather-belt beatings of Tina Turner are legend, while Rihanna was famously left black and blue by Chris Brown. Nearer home, in the glitzy corridors of Bollywood, it's whispered that Salman Khan didn't pull any punches with Aishwariya.

In fact, in India an alleged 70 per cent of women are regularly abused by their husbands. Underprivileged women, you might think, but women get knocked around regardless of how many degrees they have or the money they bring home. Domestic abuse is a funny old business for a middle-class Indian woman. You pretend it's not happening while it is. Family and friends are unbelievably blind to bumps and bruises because they dare not rock their genteel world with the admission it could happen to them.

Indian lawyer Flavia Agnes whose husband abused her for many years – breaking her bones, humiliating and starving her, and more, only found the courage to write about it decades later. She now campaigns tirelessly for abused women, knowing how hellish but also how difficult to leave that situation can be.

Similarly, Apple engineer Neha Rastogi endured emotional and physical violence from her Silicon Valley CEO husband Abhishek Gattani for a decade before she took her complaint to the US police. She had with her a phone recording of her husband humiliating and hitting her, as he routinely did. He was handed the minimum punishment, an abysmally small thirty-day custodial sentence in return.

It was for me too an unlikely situation to find myself in – an educated Bengali girl with a successful career. I couldn't even admit it to myself till the hospital run happened once too often.

Dial M for Murder

The abuse takes so many different forms. Cruelty is not just beatings after all, it goes hand in hand with a whole range of psychological, sexual and socio-economic mistreatment. In the European Union, one in five women have been sexually assaulted by a companion. One in seven women in the UK suffer severe emotional abuse at their partner's hands. And a monstrous 90 per cent of women in Pakistan are subjected to some form of mistreatment at home, from physical and sexual violence to economic deprivation.

I've known them all. After that first Christmas, George busied himself with making life difficult for me in various ways. First, of course, was the revelation of the deep debt we were in. Not disclosed till after our marriage, at which point I had already inherited it. His job was not the fancy post he'd pretended it was. And the house was tiny. The Jaguar though, would have to be kept at all cost. Bringing up our costly car, one of many contentious topics, usually ended with my ribs, cheek or throat feeling utterly and inexplicably (or that's what I told everyone else) sore.

I abandoned plans of getting the media job I was suited to and took a role in a call centre. I didn't stay long, moving on to a communications job within two months (if only to disprove that Indians belonged in call centres!), but I still remember the deprivation of those days. Every penny I had went on his toys. I had to beg and borrow, but I drew the line at stealing. I can recall the afternoon I took the last pound out of my bank account because we needed to buy food and it wasn't even the end of the month.

Then there was the isolation. Already cut off from family and friends because I'd moved halfway across the world to be with him, George ensured I didn't make any new ones either. If his friends invited us, he might take me out the first time to gauge their reactions to me; and he was far more interested in male reactions. I remember an evening that had seemed particularly successful. I had laughed, chattered and sparkled after a long, long time. At the end of the night, one of the men had leaned across and said to him, 'You must bring your beautiful wife with you again.' That was the last time I saw them. And I believe it was the last he mixed with them as well. I did make my own friends eventually, and they were the saving of me, but before that there were so many other things that wore me down.

The lies, for example. He lied about everything. It was second nature. But then I would stumble upon the truth and we'd have a blazing row. As we went along and the hitting increased, I stopped questioning him, but it made me permanently anxious. And when I say permanently, I mean even today. What made me even more of a nervous wreck was that I didn't know from one day to the next where I stood with him. Gone was the early devotion. Now it was a constant yo-yoing between 'you're too good for me' to 'you're the worst thing that's ever happened to me (but I still won't let you go)'.

Like a Hydra-headed monster, if I grappled to the ground one manifestation of his mistreatment, another would spring up and attack me. Playing out alongside the violence, orchestrated isolation, death threats, humiliations, scapegoating, and financial skulduggery, was rape. In the UK, more than half of all sexual assault victims are raped by partners and in India, in 2011, one in every five Indian men surveyed admitted to forcing their wives into sex. And it's done with impunity in countries like India, Saudi Arabia and Afghanistan, because it's still not considered a crime here.

It's one of those things women are intensely unsure about labelling, because if you're not being punched at the same time, you're never really sure it's rape. He is my husband after all, you tell yourself. I am often not in the mood, you think. If he insists on it but I don't fight (though I don't respond either), is it rape? If I am in discomfort for days after from semi-forced penetration, is *that* rape? But I didn't ask these questions till I had finally filed for divorce. Then the lawyer I'd put my query to said to me with a gleam in his eye that immediately put me off, 'Yes, it is, would you like to pursue the matter? It will, of course, put the verdict back by several months.' And a lot more money in his pocket, no doubt.

Many have to deal with much worse. Rape, even marital rape, can be so brutal as to not leave anyone in any doubt that it's happening. And then there are the women who lose their lives at the hands of their partners. On average, seven women are killed by their partners every month in England.

In India, that already frightening figure rises to one every hour, as stated before.

As one of those who got away, I can only call myself a very lucky woman. But this isn't because the establishment lifted a finger to help me. The lawyer I mentioned I did not finally engage, as he and his ilk were prohibitively expensive. And none of the organizations I reached out to could be bothered to assist either. In the last stages of the marriage, I remember calling a helpline that handed down some trite advice in a bored voice. It was a dark, winter night and I was in fear for my life, which was nothing new. I ran to the house of the neighbour I knew but they weren't in, so I had to walk back into the eye of the storm: our tiny home reverberating with the sounds of my husband's rage and threats. I shut our unlockable bedroom door behind me, jamming it with the top of a chair wedged under the door handle. I read through the night till the sun rose, and counted myself lucky once again to have survived.

Very little is done to help women in domestic abuse situations. It remains a grey area in most countries and the police, hospitals and women's charities seem not to know how to deal with it. A million calls of domestic distress are made to the British police every year, but only 45 per cent result in an arrest. In India, where there is a raft of laws, boards and bodies set up to tackle domestic violence, it continues to rise – up 27 per cent since 2012.

And there is enough anecdotal evidence around the world of the ineffectuality of social services and social workers in dealing with the same. Would the unnamed British woman attacked with a claw hammer by her sex offender ex-partner have survived if the police had acted on her complaints? Would Sunita in India have gone through as much if she'd been supported in leaving her violent husband instead of being told, 'You should have let him kill you. Life away from your husband is meaningless.'[27]

Is it any wonder so few women come forward? If they are not supported when they 'come out', they are signing their death warrant. And that's just one of many reasons women remain with their tormentors, some of them all their lives. They may have nowhere else to go, or have children they think they need to put first, not realizing that kids are better off away from abusive fathers. There are also financial reasons that hold women back. That was one of the reasons it took me four long years to make my escape.

The others were psychological and societal, as with so many other women: crippling fear, a deep lack of confidence, pathological denial, profound embarrassment and so on. Sometimes though, something happens that propels you out of that door. A switch is thrown; a light comes on and you snap out of the trance you've been in. That's what happened to me.

The Human Stains

George was not really cut out for hard work. Or so he said. So he took a job that paid less at another office. Strangely, this seemed to require longer hours, which he started putting in regularly, and happily. The overtime soon extended to overnight stays, though no extra money came in. On his last birthday with me, he called to say he wouldn't be coming home. He then hung up and was unreachable after. I spent the night sitting up, worried sick.

My career in the meantime had taken off. I was in a communications job I enjoyed, which took me travelling. A month after his alarming birthday non-appearance, I took up a weekend assignment in London. The situation with him was worse than ever when he was around, but he was no longer at home that much. I came home happier than I'd been in a long time (and earlier than planned), only to step through the door and realize something was wrong.

I walked into the kitchen as if in a dream. Or should I say nightmare? Everywhere, there was evidence of activity of the nature that little house hadn't seen in years. Flowers in a vase. Empty wine bottles on the table. The remnants of a fancy meal that my husband would not have usually had. Unless someone had urged him. Someone he wanted to impress. I hadn't been that person to him in a long while.

In the same trance-like state, I found my way to our bedroom, and there the evidence was incontrovertible and stomach-turning. Candles, more wine bottles, used tissues and a torn condom packet. I thought I might throw up. I had been scrupulously faithful to him despite opportunities with interested and sympathetic men and in spite of everything he'd put me through in those four years. With a tremulous hand, I overturned the covers on the bed to find the most vilely stained sheets. I ran to the bathroom and threw up.

A confrontation was unavoidable when he came home. The whole sorry story of infidelity and deception soon tumbled out, and I announced my intention to seek a divorce. He was penitent and nasty in turns. It no longer mattered though. I felt sick to the stomach still but euphoric at the same time. I thought I was finally free. But it was far from over. Despite friends urging me to go away with them, I could only leave our home at the risk of losing it forever, because when it comes to property, possession is nine tenths of the law. It did not house good memories but I recognized that it would be the launch pad for my resurrection. I would need to keep the house for both practical and psychological reasons.

Psychologically, it would do me no end of good to wrest it from him and practically, it would mean I could keep my steadily improving career, my hard-won circle of friends, my new life in my new country. I would not run back to India defeated by this man. But that last phase of my life with him was a test of my mettle more than at any other time. Yet I'm now glad it was, because it restored my faith in myself.

Through complex financial and legal transactions, most of which I conducted myself, I bought the house from him, and I know he never expected me to be able to do that. I paid for it too, not only more money than it was worth because he was determined to squeeze every last penny from me, but with many sleepless nights of anxiety. It's impossible to sleep when your would-be-murderer is on the floor below, and I wasn't being paranoid; George had made it clear he would kill me if things didn't go his way. One week, he stole money from my bag, leaving me with none for food even. Friends were more than happy to feed me though.

He didn't want to hand over the keys or move out but in the end he had to. I triumphantly shut the door behind him one last time and then, having learnt how to change locks from yet another trusted friend, I changed every lock in the house. Two weeks later he called to say it was over with his mistress, and would I take him back? I have never hung up more gleefully on anyone.

I lost weight. I cut my hair. I started looking like Channel [V]'s Bureau Chief again. Looking around me, I noticed that Sheffield itself had changed in that time. Concrete monstrosities were being pulled down. Sunshine was filtering through the gaps they were leaving. Beautiful new spaces were being created, with soaring girders, glass and lush greenery. This was not the city of my 'lost years' any more. This was an extension of the new-old me. Confident, attractive and full of life. The arc of abuse was complete.

Those of us lucky enough to get to the other side do come out stronger and surer than those who've never been through it. But what a price to pay. So many years lost and much else besides. To never again have the peace of mind you once had is hard to bear, even if you can barely remember what that state felt like. And the emotional baggage you carry around ever after subtly (and sometimes not so subtly) affects every subsequent relationship you have. But if I had not taken this tortuous path to get to the woods, would I be where I am now? With a wonderful new man (well, twelve years new), and the beautiful children we've made together. In the loveliest forest in England. Within touching distance of happily ever after.

8

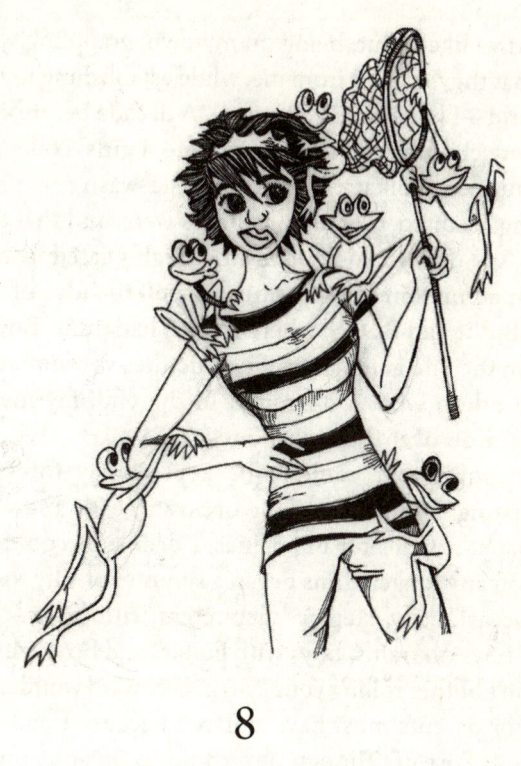

Kiss a Few Frogs

Did I go off men after my experiences with George? Did the knocking about knock my interest in them out of me? Sadly, no. I was in no hurry to settle down with another man, but I wasn't averse to being romanced. And suddenly there seemed to be a snaking line of suitors (more like un-suitors, for what they had in mind) and my ridiculous inability to walk away from men kicked in. I was thirty-one, had been round the block fully at least once and knew my way around better than

I would've liked. But, being on my own, grappling with men and what they wanted from me, while establishing my place in the world – I had done it all before. A decade before, in Delhi.

After school, I had chosen to go to a girls' college run by Irish nuns in Kolkata. Loreto College wasn't in a decrepit building, as many Calcuttan colleges were, and that appealed to me. The derelict look of another highly rated institution I had got admission to was putting me off the idea of studying there. But it had BOYS, where Loreto had nuns. Boys versus nuns on the one hand, but solid structures vs crumbling ones, on the other; what a dilemma! In the end, my instinct for survival won over the sexual one.

Of course that couldn't be kept at bay forever. After sublimating my interest in the opposite sex in the writing of newspaper articles for big dailies, I decided I couldn't really put it off any longer. Thus began a summer of silly, sweet, and very occasionally, steamy encounters with boys – boys on buses, boys on trains, boys with guitars and boys with chains.

Don't bother rolling your eyes heavenward wondering what my poor parents must have suffered because I had maternal sanction. Sort of. Though never told to do so explicitly, my mother had said often enough that women should get about a bit before they were married (peevishly, as she'd never done it herself, meeting and marrying my father early). And I intend to tell my kids just that. That premarital sex is an absolute must for figuring out love, commitment and kids; the trinity that forms the bedrock of a great many lives. So kiss a few frogs, why don't you, before you settle on just the one lily pad with a prince amongst frogs? In fact, every one of us should have a four-point frog plan.

1. Date the frog. If there's no chemistry, lose the frog. Life is too short to waste on frogs that don't float your boat.

2. Kiss the frog. If it feels right in every way (we all have different boxes we want ticked; make sure they do get ticked though), then take him to your lily pad. Or accompany him to his, but don't forget your pond-life survival strategies. You WILL need them. Because beware, bottom feeders abound.
3. The frog that comes through step two with leaping colours is no longer a frog but a prince: your Prince/Princess Charming! But if you're squeamish about toad-tossing, at least make sure you kiss (and a lot more) the frog you mean to marry before you say aye. Because do you really want slack in the sack for a lifetime?!
4. Now you really need to move in to his/her lily pad. Or have them stay at yours as often as possible. You will then have established compatibility in the only sensible way, with a dry run at living together (astrological charts just don't cut it, mausis). And I'm not talking positions (would be a *wet* run then, wouldn't it?), though why not find out what works best for you in that department too?

I didn't begin with positions. In fact, I didn't get to positions at all. I started, at sixteen, with my first grown-up kiss ever. The kind that involves tongues and, in my case, a boy with a beard. A proper Captain Haddock beard which was admirable in a school boy. Before Loreto College and being lumped with nuns, which led to encounters with boys off buses and trains, the first kiss happened in the summer while I was still at school.

He had brought his guitar. Our house was in the process of being renovated. Bang, rattle, crash, wump. The one oasis of calm where we could take his strumming and the song he'd composed for me was my parents' bedroom. There, perched on the bed, talking oh-so-seriously about music (as men with guitars AND men with beards do), he swooped down for a kiss. I was surprised, I was flattered, I was tickled by his beard. It was a delicious little secret to hug to myself and I did, but discovering the pure physical thrill of a kiss that's long and heated, which melts your innards and amazingly your bra straps, the latter falling away from you without your ever touching them, came a few years after.

It was not the bearded boy this time. Life had moved on. I had been through another one or two dissatisfyingly tepid sort-of relationships (you know the type: fellow talks endlessly about himself before he lunges for your hand and gives it a bruising squeeze as if it were the ultimate in romance), and yearned for something more ... oh I don't know ... something that soared! The first boy that came along was a man. And he was riding a bus, not a horse. His name was Something Bihari and he was, how shall I put this kindly, rustic. But a real gentleman. We spoke when he vacated his bus seat for me, tiny and tottering under many British Council books on the way home from college. Then, egged on by his friends, he mustered up the courage to ask for my number, which, much to the consternation of mausis everywhere, I gave him. Chaste I was not planning to be forever. Said Bihari chappie, however, was not destined to be my un-chaste-r either.

We went on a couple of dates where we ate strange food (pulau, he pressed upon me, and Chinese lemon chicken), lightly seasoned with awkward conversations. He bought me gifts of dire music I wished I could give back. After the third date, as he dropped me off at our gate, he leaned in for a kiss. Despite his faults, he was not bad looking and he smelt nice enough. So, as his lips touched mine, I felt a tingle. For a brief moment, I shut my eyes and lost myself in it. He was not my Prince Charming but he was not an altogether unpleasant frog.

But the moment was gone before it had even started. A loud 'ei' broke the silence and whatever tenuous magic there was in that kiss. I looked up dazedly at the source of the exclamation. It was my mother leaning out of a first floor window. My mother again, interrupting another moment of sexual discovery, though she claimed later that that wasn't what she'd meant to do. She thought she'd seen a burglar. Two of them in a clinch by the gate? Just before they stole the gate post?

The real panty-dampening stuff happened when I met a man on a train. I was twenty, on the verge of finishing college, and looking forward to a less-cloistered existence after my years at nun-run Loreto. I had decided that this expansion of my horizons should be geographical too, and had taken myself to Delhi to explore the possibilities of living and working there. It looked promising. I made it through to the last round of exams for a place in a sought-after post-graduate course.

Also, and far more interestingly for me, I was invited back for another round of interviews at a rising television production company. And I was assured, with a straight face, that living and working in Delhi would be a cakewalk for a young, single woman without a speck of street smarts. That didn't turn out to be the case, but we'll get to that. First, my adventure on the train. As it's the only one I've had in a moving vehicle, it's worth telling (but Mile High Club, here I come).

I was on a long train journey alone for the first time, heading back to Kolkata. My parents had finally allowed me this freedom. I was in a three-tier sleeper. Anyone familiar with Indian railways will know how this works. The middle tier isn't set up during the day and everyone squeezes into the bottom row to sit, eat and unfortunately, pick their noses and poke the same into other people's business. At night, the middle tier comes down and you can escape to it, but only to lie wedged like a squished aloo between slices of unappetizing parantha. And as bland as that sounds, it proved to be a very different experience for me.

The boy had been eyeing me for a while from the other end of the berth. Then he manoeuvred himself to a place beside me, and struck up a conversation. He was a smooth talker. He was attractive in a stocky Punjabi way, but he did wear the most awful gold chain, chunky and shiny. The chain ceased to matter as I found myself responding to him in the most primal way I'd ever known. We were squeezed together in our crowded compartment, rubbing against each other, sweating on each other too, but for the first time it wasn't unpleasant.

After dinner, with the lights dimmed and people nodding off, he asked to slip into my cramped middle tier with me. The train was taking me back to the nuns of Loreto in the morning, and the rebel in me wanted to do something they would have totally disapproved of. I had to decide quickly, and I chose the path of adventure. I let him lie next to me with his chest against my breasts for a while. Then his legs wound around mine, and I felt *it*, I think, in a way, for the first time. A large, hard object pressed against my tummy. This is not a torch, I thought like the little girl I still really was. But I rather liked it and didn't recoil. When his mouth came down on mine seconds later, I discovered I liked the funny, slidey, in-and-out thing he did with his tongue too. He trailed that tongue down to the dip between my breasts and found he could go no further. So, his hands found my bra clasp and unhooked it.

But the click of that clasp shook me out of my schoolgirl

fantasy of sexual liberation and dangerous living. It also alerted me to the presence of the person in the bunk below us, who was definitely awake and very possibly listening. I shushed the boy who seemed more carried away than I was. We stopped and lay still, not touching, not saying a word. Almost not breathing. Just looking at each other, though all we could see in the dark of an Indian train racing over miles of track in the dead of night were the anxious whites of our eyes. Then. Well, then, I must have fallen asleep. Because I woke by myself in the morning. It was early and still shadowy. Looking around, I found him fast asleep, back in his own bunk across the aisle. My stop was the next one. We had talked of exchanging numbers and keeping in touch. I didn't wake him, slipping away when my station came.

But Delhi I would go back to. I got the job with the television company. It was a dream role for a writer with a flair for visuals. I moved to Delhi in an excited, breathless rush with a single suitcase and even less of a plan. And my mom claimed ever after that that was when her hair turned grey (though it had been going that way a good while).

Delhi was shinier than Kolkata, and unfamiliar, with a whiff of danger about it. Little did I know how real that danger was. And what living alone on that forlorn frontier (certainly for single women) entailed. But the danger came in the shape of landlords and property touts, nosey male servants, and public transport drivers.

Delhi's male professionals seemed safe enough with their predictable expectations of, and hang-ups about, women. There was the usual need for pallidity and purity in women, but not from the ones they only meant to bed. And to me, they were only marginally more exciting than their Bengali counterparts, and only because they were a tad more alien.

After Loreto, it was quite a shock to find my life full of men of all shapes and sizes (I wish I could say interests, but their interests were all the same). Besides the Pujabis, Biharis and UPites, there were Odiyas, Mallus, Marathis and Tamils, Englishmen and Scandinavians too, including one called Lemon Rotten. Truly. Each ever so slightly more exotic than the last. And so many of them, so very keen.

It was raining men but *not* hallelujah because this turned out to be rather complicated in what was then a terribly conservative city. Delhi was heaving with young people from all over the country and hormones were on the boil, but the rules of engagement were strictly twelfth century and punishment for those who flouted them often severe. So, when an Odiya colleague drove me back after an evening out, ending up at his home when I clearly remembered asking to be dropped back at mine, I could not, even if I wanted to, 'just do it' as Nike might have advised. I had to be very firm yet wilting and Victorian instead, and insist he took me back to my own pad and left me to myself.

Another time my clean-cut Kannadiga housemate took me to see *Four Weddings and a Funeral*, but under the mistaken impression that my acceptance of his offer qualified as an invitation to *him* to come on to me. Once again it fell to me, the woman, and the recipient of the unsolicited attentions, to put an end to the situation with as little bruising to his ego as possible. Remember how it works here, I gently reminded him. Consider, I said to him, that it would really ruin our evening if we were set upon by a lynch mob. This vision of the movie audience turning upon us in fury finally dampened his ardour enough for him to leave me to focus on the more interesting Hugh Grant for the rest of the show.

But if the brushes with the opposite sex were tiresome,

tied up in socially devised knots and sometimes the stuff of nightmares (but that's another chapter!), they are unavoidable for those of us not in the running to be ascetics, because we are biologically wired to engage with prospective partners. And if we're going to engage, we might as well tangle. That tangling should be premarital and plentiful, for those looking to settle down.

I didn't have nearly enough premarital sex and therefore, made some pretty huge mistakes. Mistake, singular. I'm thinking George, of course. He was huge (okay, not huge. But thrice my size) and a big mistake. If you paid attention to the last chapter, you'd know just how much. The fact is, had I got down and dirty more often, I would've been slicker at spotting the down and the dirty.

Having said that, premarital sex is almost impossible to have in most countries, especially if you are a woman. A Pew Research Centre study on global morality in 2014 found that 90 per cent of 'predominantly Muslim nations' like Indonesia, Saudi Arabia, and Pakistan strongly disapproved of, and often punished, practitioners of premarital sex. And in the US, as late as 2003, Gallup discovered that 14 per cent thought premarital sex morally wrong (though to be fair, a good 58 per cent didn't, which was up by 5 per cent from the previous year: a Galluping improvement).

In our own Mahaan Bharat, you'd be hard put to engage in consensual premarital sexual relations with another adult, except in the most surreptitious and demeaning manner: cloak and dagger manoeuvres, hole-in-the-wall hotels, assumed identities and pretend-marriages to dupe parents, landlords, marauding policemen and the like. A live-in couple I knew in Delhi never stopped thanking their lucky stars they shared the same last name.

Another couple in Chennai went through an elaborate charade to fool their landlord, as there was no other way for them to get a place together. Naturally, it fell upon the woman to do a lot of the acting. She had to wear that ugly red stain on her head and those grotesque bits of bling married Hindu women feel the need to bear (yes bear, like a burden, not wear). As the woman bumped into the landlord and his family more often, it was she who had to lie through her teeth on a regular basis. And the man, for the price of an occasional light-hearted fib or two, got to eat his cake and have it too. You might have a pinch more freedom in showbiz, media and the microscopic intelligentsia, but how small a part of India is that? It's a well-known fact that it's better to be a cynical bigamist in Bollywood than to live unmarried with someone you love. Better to break the law than a taboo. Ask 'Garam Dharam', why don't you.

A few years ago, a Delhi court declared live-in relationships 'immoral' and 'an infamous product of Western culture'[28]. Never mind that Indians have been around and reproducing prodigiously for donkey's years, long before either the institution of marriage or western society existed. The wise judge presiding over a fast-track court dealing with sexual offences against women proved his credentials for the job further when, while exonerating a man of rape, he said, 'When a grown-up, educated and office-going woman subjects herself to sexual intercourse with a friend or colleague, she does so at her own peril. She must be taken to understand the consequences of her act. She must understand that she is engaging in an act which not only is immoral but also against the tenets of every religion. No religion in the world allows premarital sex.' Not for women at any rate, he should have added.

And if the clueless courts blunder into sense occasionally, our sagacious patriarchal society seeks to reverse what little good's been done. In 2010, the Indian Supreme Court dismissed *twenty-three* 'public decency infringement' cases against the actress Kushboo for her outspoken (and necessary) defence of a woman's right to premarital sex in India. The same court ruling upheld the right of unmarried couples to live together[29]. In 2015, this was strengthened by another Supreme Court edict that gave 'continuously cohabiting' unmarried couples the right to inherit each other's property[30]. That didn't change the fact that live-in relationships remained severely frowned upon. And premarital sex to test the waters? What were the chances Indian society would suddenly welcome those? That parents would rush to tell their sons and daughters they could now explore every part of who they were, including their sexuality, *especially* their sexuality, so when they settled they knew they were with the right person? I fancy they fretted and fumed and said 'bakwas' far too many times, and reminded the next generation that whatever the courts might say, exploring the world and finding yourself was never going to be an option.

And that's not all the GUMs (grumpy old men) and the old aunties have to say about the devilish, disgusting, depraved practice of loving someone you haven't yet married. They will warn you of:

1. Totaaal social breakdown. It starts with a kiss and before you know it, you've led your family, community and country to rack and ruin. Under mushroom clouds of destruction, buildings collapse and flames leap out from the earth's entrails to devour us. But you, you just carry on kissing your girl/guy, don't you, you malignant Mephistopheles.

2. What will happen to your family's good name? Yes, *that* good name, synonymous with child labour in your own home, bigotry of every kind outside it, and delusions of grandeur. *That* good name. What will happen to it when you taint it with the horror that is premarital sex?
3. Who will marry you? Now that you've loved someone you weren't told to and expressed that love physically as you're designed to do, who on earth will marry you? Certainly not any of the fine men and women the mausis picked for you, cast from the same mould that created those doyennes of doom. And without marriage (especially if you're a woman), what will you be? Nothing.
4. You will catch horrible diseases leading to a protracted and painful death. Well, not from kissing you won't. But from sleeping around you might. Too much love *can* kill you. But there is an alliterative answer to your problem: caution, condoms and canny exits (when safety is an issue).
5. Finally and most importantly, it is not Indian! It only takes the slightest misstep to make you 'Un-Indian', as I found on my return from the Philippines. It could be speaking up for yourself, or wearing shorts in the heat long before you're even a woman and can be considered 'looj'. Or it could be unsanctioned kissing and canoodling. Now that's just off the Richter Scale of Un-Indianness, and gotta be punished. Because we're NOT like this only. Although we did write the Kama Sutra but ho-hum-ahem, let's forget about that.

What part of unattached people who feel for each other, wanting to feel each other, is a slap in the face of Indian society? In Mumbai in 2015, police raided hotels, dragging out lovers to humiliate and upbraid. That's right, people legally going about their business, unlike the police! And although the latter cited Section 110 – indecent behaviour in public – as the basis for their arrests, each of these forty couples had, in fact, been in private rooms. This is no isolated incident either, with hundreds of instances of assault, extortion, humiliation and incarceration of unmarried lovers by the police as well as the moral police every year in India.

Said one of the women rounded up in the Mumbai raid after she was slapped by a policewoman when she refused to pay the fine, 'Do we have freedom as citizens of India? How can you fine and demean us and intrude into our privacy? Making love to the person of my choice in a private room doesn't amount to indecent behaviour in public.'[31] Much of the time, the law is plainly not being broken, but even if it is, do these archaic edicts from 1860 have a leg to stand on today? Petting in public may have seemed 'indecent' back when legs were demurely draped, but swamped by bodacious hoardings, bootilicious male magazines and bountiful porn as we are these days, something as mild and indeed, sweet, as PDA simply cannot be deemed offensive.

Premarital sex (public or otherwise) is also the sensible thing to do. Nothing in life is guaranteed, but there are trials for jobs, test runs for cars and pilots for TV shows allowing us to try before we buy. To sample before we settle. Why should we be any less practical with the Mother of All Decisions (for most of us)? We build lives on choices made largely on the basis of our sexual urges. The most important decision many of us make is who we sleep with long-term, which then becomes the foundation for everything else – families, careers and social engagement. Don't we need to be allowed to explore our sexual options well enough to get it right? Statistics can be manipulated to prove that both premarital abstention and premarital cohabitation lead to blissful, unbroken marriages depending on the surveyor's religious persuasion. So, with Mark Twain, we can assume they are *all* 'damned lies' and trust common sense and experience instead. We know, for example, that marrying someone we know well, warts and all, makes us more realistic about what we're taking on. Which in turn makes it work better.

I've married twice (with a divorce in between, thanks). The first time I got married, I really didn't know the man well, Biblically or otherwise. Nor did I know him long enough, or whether he was long enough, i.e., whether we would fit well together sexually. Therefore, my first marriage, based on a romantic fiction, failed. The second one, built on a great many wonderful things but also an intimate knowledge of each other gathered over the months before our marriage, continues to thrive (fingers crossed). Because a happy marriage is a sexually satisfied marriage and finding a good fit is essential.

In India, many young men and women are forced to become bedfellows and life partners when they've barely laid eyes on each other, with unhappy consequences. Domestic abuse and dowry deaths are more frequent in such situations. Dr Ramani Sundaresan, a Delhi-based psychotherapist, is not surprised because, in her words, 'nobody tells the wife that the man has a bad temper or abusive parents.'[32] And if divorce rates are lower, what of it? Do the people involved really have the option of walking away from these travesties? What of happiness, which is not about whether you're still shackled together at a 109, but the good times you've had along the way. And the frogs you've kissed. Or even that *one* frog you've kissed again and again and thoroughly enjoyed.

Without the chance to explore our sexuality, we may never discover what we are drawn to, till it's too late. Till we've been pushed into an unworkable marriage and a whole brace of lives have been ruined as a result. Amongst other things, we get to find out if we like the same or the opposite sex. A lady doctor in Delhi committed suicide recently while outing her homosexual husband who hadn't revealed this rather important fact to her *before* they married. So, the wife ends up dead after years of heartache, and the man is arrested ostensibly for making dowry demands, but it could just as well have been for violating section 377[33].

Section 377 is yet another dodgy British law from 1860 (what a good year that was for bigotry). It criminalizes 'sex against the order of nature' which the British themselves have outgrown but we faithfully cling to, even though it may be against our earliest tenets. 600 people were arrested for contravening section 377 in 2014, up from 150 in 1996. Well, congratulations, we're getting more 'Indian' all the time! And people are dying. How differently it might have turned out for that couple and a thousand others if he had not felt compelled to hide his homosexuality. And in some cases, if they'd even known. How many young Indians know for sure what their sexual orientation is without the opportunities to find out? One shamefaced and frightened encounter, as had by a friend who told me he was confused for years after, does not certainty make.

Most of all, it is young women who need to have premarital sex. Lots of it. Not so much due to a biological need (but why not that too?) but for the good of the world. Yes, really. A world that allows women to make choices for themselves, sexual and otherwise, that allows them to figure out what they need in order to make life work for them and their families, does itself a favour. Empowered women make sexual choices that bring down disease, increase collective wealth, produce healthier children and more stable families.

All this can be done by allowing women some nookie? Hell, yeah. But what happens instead? Double standards, that's what. In India and much of the East, although premarital sex is apparently discouraged for men too, they aren't punished for it the way women are. What, after all, are prune-faced beardy fathers actually telling their sons in private? That it's okay for them to dip their wick. But women who do so are sluts.

Yet knowing that 'sticks and stones may break their bones, but words will never hurt them,' they decided in some parts of the world to put sexually independent women to death. With stones. This evolved and humane practice is prevalent in at least fifteen countries, including Pakistan, Afghanistan and Iraq, where it is on the rise. 'Stoning is a cruel and hideous punishment. It is a form of torturing someone to death,' stated Naureen Shameem, of the human rights group, Women Living Under Muslim Laws. 'It is one of the most brutal forms of violence perpetrated against women in order to control and punish their sexuality and basic freedoms[34].' Three out of four women in prison in Pakistan are apparently there for 'unlawful sex'.

Though women don't often or legally get executed in India for the same, they are chastised enough and in different ways for it anyway, while men are let off on the grounds that boys will be boys. 'Just because India achieved freedom at midnight does not mean that women can venture out after dark. They should ensure they do not board buses with few passengers. The woman should have thought twice before boarding the suspicious private bus that night. Though the incident was condemnable, she should have behaved keeping in mind the situation,' opined Indian politician Botsa Satyanarayana on the Delhi rape of 2012[35].

But that would never have been said about a man who was butchered for having boarded a bus after midnight. Men have 'needs', you see, which excuses everything. Women don't; they have evil designs. Why else would they want to explore and develop in the same way as men? But try this on for size. If the business of love, domestic harmony and childbirth is seen as the preserve of women, if women have to keep it all going, shouldn't they be *frigging* experts at it too?

But I'm no expert either; I just like to talk about it. All sorts of things stood in the way of my becoming one – my inner schoolmarm, body-image issues, blue cloths and the wrong boys. Blue cloths, you ask? Like the green screens these days, blue cloth was used as TV show backdrops on which graphics were superimposed when we were in television. And occasionally, they became sheets to sleep under at night. Once in a blue moon, an awfully cute Mallu boy might have found himself wrapped up in one with a not entirely unattractive Bong girl, and decided to do more than sleep. Just a bit more. Followed by this conversation the next morning.

Bong girl: Um, what happened?

Mallu boy (smiling): Nothing much.

Bong girl: Oh, er, and whatever did happen ... was it okay?

Mallu boy (amused, but infinitely gentle and sensitive considering his age): It was wonderful. Why wouldn't it be, cuddling a pretty girl on a cold Delhi night?

I went back to Kolkata after that. Not because of *that*. Although indirectly, probably because of that. Because I was spending nights on the studio floor without a place to call my own. I'll tell you all about that in a bit. But I went home without the intimate knowledge of men I had hoped to have got under my belt. In my case, kissing a few frogs really did mean just kissing. It was never the right time or the right man. Or maybe it was me who wasn't right. Or ready. Or quite possibly it was the city. Shiny, sleazy, censorious Delhi. Whatever it was, I went on to Duncan and then George, completely unprepared for men and the sorrows they sometimes bring.

9
Delhi's Underbelly

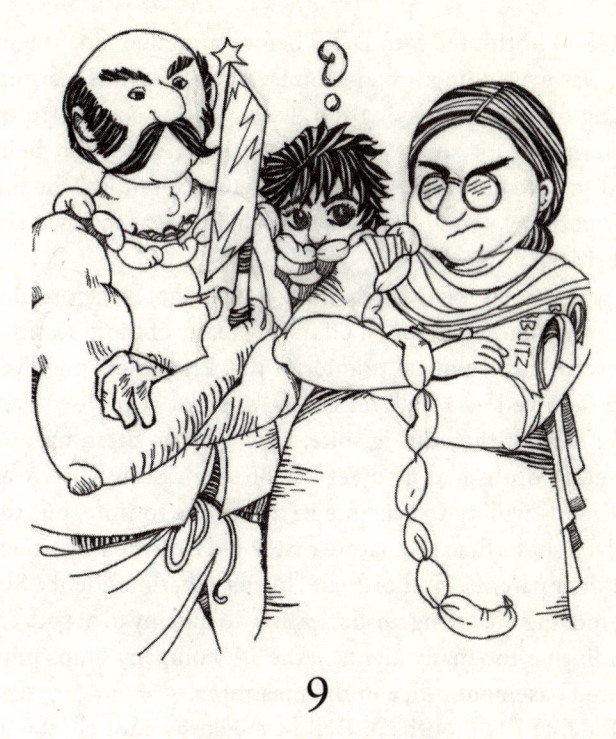

Delhi felt fleeting, though I was there for a year. And if it didn't teach me about boys, it taught me about the seamy side of life. Somewhat. Not enough to enable me to sidestep some of what was coming (Duncan, George, and er, Duncan, George) but enough to write a chapter on it years later with the feeling that I've lived some, haven't I?

The job I'd snagged was a dream. A rookie reporter job at a time when the news television boom was in the offing. Anyone my age and with my artistic propensities would kill for it. So I hotfooted it to Delhi before someone did. The job itself was everything it had promised to be – I was learning, making friends and having fun. I was writing scripts (to the consternation of some senior reporters, I was soon being asked to rewrite theirs, but shhhh, let's not remind them of it). And to my young, starry-eyed delight, I was interviewing celebrities.

I was also, supposedly, learning how to do television edits, but I must admit I dropped off during many of these sessions; they were too technical to interest me. Plus, I was massively sleep-deprived as I had yet to find a place of my own, and in the dark of the editing suite, I was able to catch up on it (the edit booths had many excellent uses). Even better were the friends willing to take me in from time to time, but that involved subterfuge of a nature that could land them in trouble with their parents, landlords and hostel superintendents. So, I kept moving on, trying unsuccessfully to find my own pad, and spending far too many nights in the TV company's mosquito-infested basement office in the meantime.

The first few months in Delhi were cushy enough, staying with family friends in a super-rich Delhi neighbourhood. But that honeymoon had to end and I was yanked out of that cosy existence into the scary world of the room-to-let racket. I first found a shared room in Alakananda, which seemed above board till I realized all was not kosher below stairs. From the duplex's subterranean kitchen where sausages were being stuffed and salami sliced for their deli business, the wrong smells were wafting out. Innocent vegetarian souls that my roomies were, they were oblivious to them, but my keen carnivorous nose sensed something fishy going on. Or the opposite of fishy. The sausage and salami meat did not smell or taste of pig or any farmyard animal I'd ever sunk my teeth into.

I was soon refusing to have any on the grounds that I'd turned vegetarian. I hadn't, but had every intention of turning sleuth. During the day though, our large landlady would position herself between the kitchen door and the passage that led to our bedrooms, reading filmi mag after filmi mag. When she did vacate her chair to make her way to the toilet, her fearsomely moustachioed manservant would take her place with his formidable arms folded in front of him, and the chance to slip into the dimly lit and foul (not fowl) smelling Kitchen of Fleshy Mysteries would be foiled.

What I hadn't expected was that while I watched them, they, especially the man, would be watching ME. I began to worry that their dark kitchen was the Delhi equivalent of Soylent Green and I was next on the menu (though none of my roommates, some of them a good bit heftier than me, had disappeared yet). But I was wrong about the nature of his interest in my flesh.

One dark night while I was alone in my room, with my roommate out necking in some back alley (and getting arrested for her pains), the odd-job man came barging in. We had the tiniest of barred windows that let little light in, and though I couldn't see him I knew who he was from his distinctive smell – a combination of unidentified flesh and the betel nut he chewed. As he approached my bed sneakily and lifted the edge of the covers, I held my breath, getting ready to dodge his knife or whatever he used to pin his prey. But then he started stroking my bare leg, and it became clear he hadn't come to make mince of me; he had quite other intentions. So I yelled. I screamed so loud it brought the house down. Down from their bedrooms on the floor above came tumbling the other paying guests. The lights in my room came on to show faces as aghast as mine. The manservant tried to brazen it out with a cock (what it's ever about) and bull story about a cat. Which seemed to be going down well with our audience when one of the women from upstairs suddenly exploded.

'You battameez cheez,' she cried, as if about to start a quawwali performance. I almost expected the other roomies to jump in with the back-up thumri. 'You snuck into my room too,' she said waggling her finger at the man. 'But there were two of us sleeping there that night and you chickened out (the only chicken then to be found in *that* kitchen, I thought). Don't you think we saw you sneaking away?!'

The mustachioed manservant deflated under the two-pronged attack, but just as we girls seemed to be winning, our landlady came steaming in like an overloaded cargo train. Next thing we knew, instead of dismissal or a dressing down for greasy Mr Moustache, WE were being shown the door. As I slung my single rucksack over my shoulder to leave the following morning, I noticed the man was making himself scarce (or had met his end in the landlady's industrial-sized meat grinder), but the lumbering landlady was guarding the kitchen entrance with an extra-scary scowl pasted on her face, just for us.

Months later, we discovered that the man had been arrested for spiriting pet dogs away from their posh south Delhi homes, and not for molestation as we might have hoped. But neither was a surprise.

I think I must have inspected more holes-in-walls than the rat catchers of Hamlyn. One was a house full of women in various states of drugging and dishabille, which was very probably a brothel. The woman I imagined to be the 'Madame' said I could share a room with one of them but in a sniffy way that suggested she didn't think I'd make her much money. I already had a career (if not a room), so I made my way to the next property.

I usually reconnoitred rooms on weekends, as weekdays were happily and far more productively spent at the television studio. At the next place, I was eagerly led to a pleasant, well-lit room by the landlord himself (a task usually delegated to the wife or servant in Delhi, who were sometimes interchangeable). I liked the look of the room but not so much the leering landlord. It struck me that I'd been brought into the room through the man's bedroom. 'And how do I let myself in or out, since I work at a television studio and keep unusual hours?' I asked, hoping to be pointed to a door leading out I hadn't noticed. 'Naaat to baather, Beti' he said, his nicotine-stained smile widening, 'you will be coming through my room but think of it as yours. I shall even wait up for you when you're late.'

I didn't wait for more.

Eventually, I found a room with a kitchenette and a shared terrace in Chittaranjan Park, the stronghold of the domiciled Bengalis of Delhi. I thought that might be a good thing, that they might embrace me (platonically for a change) as one of their own. So I moved in lock, stock and barrel, i.e., one rucksack crammed with very strange clothes (because I had yet to discover style) + a load of long johns I'd never wear (as my parents held firm to the belief that Delhi had arctic winters) + one frying pan (they also hoped I would learn to fry an egg at least).

While I looked around my new room, the reception committee of the landlord and his grown sons sized me up. From the dark interior of the house came a quavering female voice announcing the imminent dishing up of 'maach bhaat', and the younger men scuttled out. My portly landlord, in a hurry to leave as well, handed over the key with a brief (very brief, with maach waiting) lecture on the 'phaine moraaalsh' of the Bengali woman.

I could have whooped with joy. I finally had a place to stay and it wasn't too bad. But an obstacle was waiting just round the corner. Or rather, like with the last place, it was the absence of one that was a problem. There appeared to be neither lock nor handle on my side of an interconnecting door. So, I asked very nicely about arrangements to secure it from my side. And the sweet, syrupy miasma that had hung in the air suddenly turned to frost. 'Keno lagbe?' asked the patriarch testily. For security and privacy, I stated. At which he drew himself to his full five feet and said, 'Aapni ki amader chor na molestaaar dakchhen?' and without further ado (including doing anything about the door), he stormed out.

And I realised why the last girl who'd roomed there had moved in such a hurry. Had anything happened, or had the implications of a door without a lock spooked her as it did me? I had paid a deposit however, and had nowhere else to go that night. But I had a plan. In the room was a cupboard that looked flimsy enough for me to push across the floor but not so rickety it could be knocked over without ruckus or effort in the dead of night. It took me nearly an hour to move it, but I did get some sleep that night.

I woke, however, to golmaal (or three very gol maals kicking up a fuss). The Bengali bhadralok had discovered they'd been outfoxed by a pint-sized Bengali woman and weren't happy. I was sent on my way with an outraged Bong flea in my ear, and without my deposit.

I wish I'd known then about the handbook all these Delhi landlords owned, and not just landlords, but a great many men around the world. It tells them all they need to know about women (ain't much to us, y'know). The most thumbed bit is frequently the section on feminine harlotry called the SLUT Scale. S for slatternly, L for Loose, U for uninhibited, and

T for tramps. It puts forward the age-old and still firmly held belief that most women are just waiting to be invaded by man's many icky, sticky (and often stubby) protrusions.

There are, of course, degrees of decadence amongst us, but we do all figure somewhere on this global slapper index. From the totally innocent five-year-old to the eighty-five-year-old grandma who would rather find her teeth than a man, we've all managed to lure some hapless man to his doom with our uncontrollable coming-out-of-our-ears sexuality. Indian politician Vijayvargiya wisely warns women, 'Your provocative dresses are responsible for all deviations in society[36].' While Iranian cleric Hojatoleslam Kazem Sedighi thunders, 'many women who don't dress modestly lead young men astray and spread adultery in society which increases earthquakes'[37].

And if you thought such 'wisdom' was the preserve of the East, check this pearl out from American media mogul Pat Robertson, 'Feminism encourages women to leave their husbands, kill their children, practice witchcraft, destroy capitalism and become lesbians'[38]. This can't go on. No further man, beast, deeply flawed economic system or slippy-slidey tectonic plate should be endangered by our earth-shatteringly sluttish ways. But just how slutty are you?

Garden variety or Microsluts: She'll lead you up the garden path but won't let you past the front door. A tepid tease and no more, registering a mild 2.0 to 3.9 on the Harlotry Index. 'Environmental damage limited to trembling of indoor objects.' Tina Fey is our Garden Variety Slut gold standard, because she sure does provoke, but only with her abandon with words.

The 'light to moderate' practitioner of harlotry is the **Stealthy Slapper**, who, at a 4.0 to 5.9 on the SLUT Scale poses a middling hazard to mankind's health. You know her by her hint of cleavage and uncovered legs, triggering that uncontrollable frustration in men which culminates in all the sexual harassment and molestation that's about (proof that when men can't rein it in, it's not their fault). 'Can cause damage of varying severity to poorly constructed buildings'. J-Lo's our pin-up for this one: 'People equate sexy with promiscuous. They think because I'm shaped this way, I must be scandalous[39].' Of course you are, Jen, since so many boys insist.

The **Slut Major or the Slagosaurus** is an unapologetic, irredeemable harlot, who takes her pleasure where and when it suits her. They follow the gospel of Jessica Alba: 'I don't think a girl's a slut if she enjoys sex. I could have a one-night stand … and not try to make it more[40]'. An earth-shaking, burn-at-the-staking 6.0 to 7.9 on the SLUT scale, these women cause death and destruction wherever they go. 'Damage can be caused far from the epicentre. Strong to violent shaking at focal point'. Yet who really inflicts this damage to our social fabric, women asserting their sexual independence, or the men who seek to control them? It's a mystery.

But who should really come out on top with a HUMONGOUS 8 to 10 on the SLUT Scale? The sage Christina Aguilera even sang about it, 'If you look back in history it's a common double standard of society. The guy gets all the glory the more he can score while the girl can do the same and yet you call her a whore.' The average man, for a range of reasons, societal and some claim, biological, is a whole lot more wanton than the average woman. Western men have an average of seven sexual partners in their lifetime to the five for women and the gap is greater in the East. But do they ever get called those short, staccato, venom-dripping names like slut, slag or whore? Reserved for them are those mellifluous, rolls-off-the-tongue labels like Don Juan, Casanova and Lothario. Even language is unfair to women.

More seriously though, what the widespread adoption of this all-women-are-slags belief leads to are frequent sexual assaults and sexual harassment. When the old man in a packed bus rubs up against your schoolgirl derriere, you know you're being molested, regardless of how inexperienced your bottom might be. But when your co-worker leans over your desk to look down your top repeatedly, you could be left wondering whether he really needs to borrow your scissors that many times or should you ram it into his nuts instead. In much of the world, sexual harassment gets swept under the carpet constantly (rape does too except it's rather more obvious some of the time). In India, sexual harassment is bizarrely called 'Eve teasing', implying that like Eve, the woman had tempted and the man had succumbed. She'd asked for it, so, nine times out of ten, the 'teasing' goes unpunished.

I wonder if getting your dick out in a darkened office with one female colleague left in, and waving it in her face, is light teasing? Just a laugh? Well, I know the lady in question did not laugh. First, she couldn't believe her eyes, then she felt so sick she could hardly shift. When she could get her trembling legs to move, she ran like she'd never run before. She told her boss the next morning. The man was brought in, a senior executive. He denied it, and there it ended. But then it happened again. He found her alone at the end of the day and this time, in retribution, he sneaked up on her and hung it in front of her face. SHE left. Not just the company but the country. And he continued on his glorious trajectory to the top of the corporate heap.

Sexual harassment couldn't be more in-your-face than in this instance, but it comes in so many shapes, sizes, shades and degrees of ambiguity that it can leave you mightily disturbed without a smidgeon of certainty about what really happened. One in three women are sexually harassed in the workplace. On the streets around the world, it is 65 per cent of all women, of whom 71 per cent do not report it (which rises to 90 per cent in India) and only 15 per cent of those who did, felt it had been handled fairly (falling to only 5 per cent in India). Waving your unsolicited wick in a woman's face is clearly harassment (and you still get let off the hook), but there's a legion of less obvious forms of pestering that I think we should try and identify in a little game (which is all that harassment is to some men) I call *Slug, Parry, Avoid* after the odious British TV reality show '*Snog, Marry, Avoid*'.

1. Let's start with Barack Obama. An easy target, standing tall, dark and handsome in front of the whitest of white preserves – the White House. But when he said of Indian-American Attorney General Kamala Harris days before her induction, 'She's brilliant, she's dedicated, and she's tough. She also happens to be the best-looking attorney general', was he crossing the line himself?
Political commentator Amanda Marcotte certainly thought so. 'As a tool to keep women playing along with male dominance, benevolent sexism works far better than hostile sexism,' she explained. Reporter Katie J.M. Baker opined, 'Women put up with enough unsolicited attention as it is; the President doesn't need to legitimize the practice by piling on.'[41]
But were they right in this instance? He said she looked good *after* praising her brains and character. Best to not say it at all, I agree, but haven't we commented on

Mr Obama's fine figure ourselves? Haven't we warmed to Canadian Prime Minister Justin Trudeau partly because he isn't hard to look at? Plus, *how* it's said also matters. Barack Obama, I imagine, didn't deliver his compliment with a smirk and a wink and a quick feel of his crotch. And he apologized for his comment after, though in the face of a whirlwind of womanly ire, it has to be said. So in this instance, avoid, I say, by which I mean ignore. Because though Obama himself may be big fish, this particular incident is small fry in the annals of sexual harassment.

2. On then to Bill. Bill Clinton. Unlike the previous scenario, where a mildly inappropriate comment was made, the Monica Lewinsky imbroglio was a whole different mouthful. Now Clinton is one of the better presidents the US has had. He's smart, his politics are sassy, but his treatment of women is quite another matter.

He took advantage of a much younger woman in his power, drawing her into humiliating albeit consensual sexual activities (we ne'er did believe your 'I did NOT have sex with that woman' bluster, Buster). As Monica herself confirmed in *Vanity Fair* in 2014, what made it sexual harassment was not that it was forced but that she became the scapegoat for the whole sorry affair (as women do). For a situation she was half-manipulated into, she was hounded, humiliated and hung out to dry (not unlike her infamous blue dress), even by the man who had said he'd look out for her.

'I was the Unstable Stalker, the Dimwit Floozy ... the Clinton administration, the special prosecutor's minions, the political operatives on both sides, and the media were able to brand me. And that brand stuck, in part because it was imbued with power[42].' Ten years on, she's still a byword for slutty sex while Clinton has returned to his position as one of the world's most admired men. But it's not just him. Powerful men treat countless women with similar contempt. With impunity. Without consequences. Think *Tehelka* and Tarun Tejpal, or TERI's Rajendra Pachauri. They abused women in their power. What the women didn't do or felt compelled to do doesn't change that fundamental fact. So, slug. Knock 'em off their pedestals, rub their noses in the dirt a little. That's all the humble pie they're likely to taste.

3. Quite another kettle of icky fish is the little man in his dark corner of the office, skulking behind his daily rag, occasionally flashing the bared boobies on Page 3 at you. To let you know you're on his mind. Parts of you, anyway. Page 3 may be a phenomenon peculiar to Britain, but there's no dearth of the same all over the world – men's magazines, internet porn and even celebrity pages heaving with bums and breasts. Not to forget the 'item number' in India, institutionalized objectification like the British Page 3. If 'enjoyed' in seclusion, no one can have anything to say about it. When it's shoved under women's noses, draped over shared workspaces or used to send clear messages of intent, then that isn't acceptable at all. The fact is, guys, gawping at pornography in public does nothing for your chances of getting lucky (which you bizarrely, inexplicably, seem to think it might do; what are the chances Pia will whip out her breasts when she spots you peering at a paper pair?).

Studies show that when men are asked 'Would you ever consider forcing a woman to have sex?' after they've eyeballed sexualized images of women, they are more likely to answer 'yes'[43]. SLUG. There's no other way.
4. There are many more manifestations of sexual harassment. From actual touching to belittling on the basis of gender ('Aww, c'mon, you'll never be able to do that, you Little Woman') to sexist trolling ('Look what the slag's wearing on Facebook') to stalking ('She showed me the soles of her feet, clearly begging me to follow her.' No, mate, she was running away from you), there's such a vast and frightening range, that all you can do is slug, slug, slug, parry, parry, avoid, slug, parry, slug. And in real life, never ever stay shtum about it.

It's a good time to remember there are many good men too. My husband (the second one), my father, my many fabulous male friends and millions of other fine fellows out there would never raise a finger against a woman (or stick them where they don't belong). But there was a particularly chivalrous young man I wanted to tell you about. The bearded one I'd shared my first kiss with. He'd moved to Delhi around the time I was in search of a home there. Being a single man doing a post-graduate course at Delhi University, landing a shared room with another such fella proved easy enough for him. And there he stayed for the most part, immersed in academia.

Neither of us knew the other was in town. So, one winter's night, when I'd walked out of another unsuitable room, and gone looking for a friend at the university, I wasn't expecting to bump into my bearded boy of yore. Mellow after a few rounds of momos, I thought nothing of going back with him when he offered to share his narrow boys hostel bed for the night. And this, for a change, is not a cautionary tale. Because sometimes you just know what's in a person's heart. And my bearded boy had a heart of gold. As I drifted to sleep in his arms that night, fully clothed and perfectly unloverlike, I was warm, happy and ... safe. The other boys who had been sworn to secrecy played their part too. Keeping a lookout for the hostel superintendent. Forming a human hedge that I ducked behind on my way to the bathrooms that night. Food, too, was smuggled up to me in my friend's Santiniketan jhola.

Grown used to being objectified and harassed by the landlords of Delhi, the respect and bonhomie I got from my friend and his buddies that night was a joy and a relief. In the morning, he wrapped me in his warm plaid jacket as my own, he decided, was too thin for the temperatures Delhi had plunged to. When I returned to Kolkata, that jacket went with me, because the pressures of career and education had meant we hadn't managed to meet again. The jacket changed hands again and again and BB and I only ever saw it in pictures, turning up on different people over the years, and we laughed about its journey. Our own journeys took us from Kolkata to Delhi to Europe, never to meet again. But our friendship, which went from a kiss to a night of warmth and protection, blossomed into a friendship that ran deeper with every passing year, over the net though it all transpired. We became the best of virtual friends, talking daily, exchanging confidences about love, life and our troubles, which included strokes, depression and divorces. We giggled, I cried, he cheered me up. We promised to meet. Nearly every day. Till one day he travelled from his home on a day trip, slightly under the weather, and never came back again. He died of a massive organ failure whilst still in a coma, in a hospital far, far away from me.

I am still getting used to life without my dearest virtual friend – my beloved Bearded Boy.

10

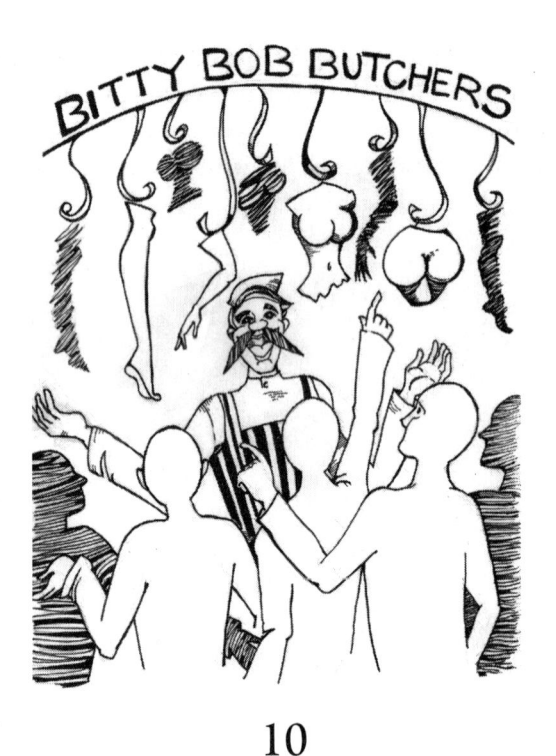

Bits and Bobs

Ten years, one failed marriage and a change of career later, having a roof over my head was the least of my problems. In fact, that was the one thing I could actually celebrate – having bought my own house in my straitened circumstances. Small though the house was, it was more than adequate for the single life I was planning to lead after my divorce, and once I'd thrown out George's faux-ostentatious tat, it became the neat little minimalist haven I had always meant it to be.

If both my marriage and my change of career had been disasters, the divorce itself – the process of scrubbing both the house and my life clean of my execrable ex-husband – was a triumph in every way. Buying the house from George involved a great deal of financial and legal mumbo-jumbo which, with my lack of funds, I had to figure out for myself. From pillar to post, from bank to bank, I went looking for the best deal for the determined-to-succeed-pauper.

In my spare time, I spent every moment doing the very arithmetic I'd hated growing up, just to make sure I could avoid loans or handouts to survive, *and* pull off the purchase of the house as well. And that's when I was not swotting up on divorce law, forced as I was to conduct my divorce myself, because I could either have a lawyer or a house. I chose house.

'Oh, you'll be charged per page of every letter or document we send to your husband', said the fifth lawyer I went to see, sounding like an echo of those before him.

'And these letters and documents to my husband will say what?' I asked, fairly sure of the answer.

'That you intend to divorce him on the grounds of irreconcilable differences, infidelity and unbearable cruelty. Variations of this really, said weekly, till the divorce actually comes through, which takes about two years on an average.'

I did not need to do the sums in my head yet again; I already knew it would cost thousands I didn't have. 'That's okay,' I said getting up, never to darken the door of a divorce lawyer again. 'I can tell him that again and again at no cost.'

The next day found me at Sheffield's grand Central Library looking into the law.

If I delved into subjects I had given a wide berth to before, I also learnt practical skills from my girlfriends I never imagined I would need, from changing locks to basic plumbing, ensuring

I would never find myself beholden to tradesmen. Or to the man next door who now thought it was his job to help me, since the husband had skedaddled, and help himself to the perks that he imagined came with me.

The whole business felt a feminist triumph. And I settled down to what I imagined would be a somewhat solitary but, for all that, a contented life. I had no idea that getting rid of 'my man' (though even the phrase in connection with him rankled) would be seen as an all-clear to every other man who knew me or those about to make themselves known to me.

At thirty, a late bloomer, I was finally coming in to season (the proof was in the pounding – the number of men pounding the pavement outside my home). Somewhere along the way I had developed a figure. The breadth of my top half had finally caught up with my bottom half and, keenly aware of how blessed I was to have a Scarlett O' Hara waistline, I could now only rejoice at this near-hour-glass figure. Curvy, if truncated (at just about five feet). I was blossoming and basking in it. But with bountiful breasts come great responsibility, if you are a feminist to boob, er, boot. It was great to have them but it was also important to be aware of all the drooling on your person that came with this new territory.

Not having had as much male attention growing up, this onrush of interest was surprising, as well as, yes, a wee bit flattering. And so, that first date with a new man came rather quickly, upsetting the self-contained life I had planned for myself – a life of rainy afternoons reading, pots of hot chocolate with friends in snug city-centre cafes, and experiments with cooking and clothes that involved exotic new ingredients like teriyaki sauce and tube tops. It seemed a good plan, with the occasional twinge of unhappiness that the family I grew up with was far away, and a little family of my own, far in the future, if at all.

But I didn't want anything to happen too soon either. I really didn't think it would, not with all the stories in magazines about divorcees who search the earth for love ever after and my own circles' mournful tales of the lack of 'talent' out there. No matter. I was out for nothing more than a drink and a laugh. Yet, as we know, men are like sheep and if one comes along, others are bound to follow. I think of them as Kolkata mini-buses (which I'm more familiar with than sheep), all hurtling towards you at the same time, or none at all to be seen. But let's go with the animal metaphors. Soon, I had a snaking queue outside my front door of men of all ages, sizes, colours and shapes. No kidding. The one time I wanted a relatively man-free life, along came a multitude (like Kolkata buses again, see).

I looked out the window one wintry morning, not more than a month after the start of my single life, and groaned. They had pitched tents (okay, I am kidding this time, but one *had* threatened to do so if I refused to go out with him). So, despite my best intentions, I found myself in the game again. I was soon picking through the offerings, discounting the depraved, diseased or dangerous straight away. Or so I thought.

Andrew was from London. He seemed clever, chirpy and not cheap (in that he bought me mocha latte in our office canteen every chance he got; after George, that was practically princely). He asked me out and I said yes, thinking it might be fun; with similar politics and reading habits, we had plenty to talk about. He had a compelling Cockney charm about him too. I was also dimly aware that he liked hovering behind me quite a lot. If I felt eyes on my booty, I could be fairly sure I'd turn and see Andy beaming at 'me behind'.

Despite my enjoyment of my new-found body confidence, this close scrutiny of my bottom did bother me a tad. Still, I didn't know if I wasn't being too sensitive (aren't all women assailed by such doubts?). So off we went on a date I hoped would be a quiet evening of convivial conversation and good food. Instead, I found myself in a cocktail bar where the din and bustle made a good chinwag impossible. And the bar stools! So strangely positioned that I spent most of my time leaning over, no, nearly falling over, to reach my drink. Andy, however, seemed elated with how the evening was going, his flushed cheeks and glazed eyes attested to his having had either too much food, alcohol, or as it transpired ... bottom.

'Honestly? You didn't know he took you there so he could watch your bottom go up and down on that stool, mimicking ...'

'Enough, enough,' I said to my friend Carla, choking on the previous night's meal as it came rushing up.

Needless to say, I didn't go out with Andy again, but it was a most educational date. A whole new world of men was laid bare before me. A world I hadn't really been aware of. My girlfriends were more than happy to bring me up to speed. Turned out Andy was a Bob, a Bitty Bob. Bitty Bobs are men who are fixated on certain parts of a woman rather than the whole. More nastily known as Meathook Men, they have made objectification a fine art, drilling down to a small section of a woman to lust after, to the exclusion of all else.

Bitty Bobs may be Breast Men, Ass Men and even Bush Men (like their namesake, they bear pointy spears when lost in undergrowth). They are extremely rigid with their down-to-the-nth-detail body proportion preferences. And even amongst them, there are sub-classes ('sub' being the operative word). The Breast Men, for example, like them big, but some are dead set on a Double D, even when droopy, while others pine for perky. Equally, you'd never find the Big Ass Men hanging with the Tiny Tush Toms. The world of Bitty Bobs is narrow (in every sense) and divided by disagreements about what's best. Hilarious on the face of it, these fixations on women's body parts are a particularly unsavoury form of sexism. And though I might have woken up to it fully in Britain, this persistent, pernicious objectification of women happens ALL. OVER. THE. WORLD.

There are many (many, many) Bitty Babus in India, but like with all things sexual, they keep this under wraps, under the starched dhoti, checked lungi, peekaboo mundu, etc. What these men, Bobs and Babus, are doing is dismembering women in their heads, claiming a part of their bodies while binning the rest as unimportant, like cuts of meat at a butcher's. So, we become less important than a live cow and only as much as its dead bits. Oh, men are judged on looks too, but only women are mentally dissected, weighed up on the merits of individual parts and assigned their worth as human beings on that basis. Bob is also bitty because he has an itty-bitty brain (and maybe an itty-bitty you know what, but let's not descend to their level), so you can bet he'll bleat resentfully, 'But women tell us all the time that they check out our asses, our pecs, even our nails!' We are checking to see if you're clean enough to let into our homes, and maybe, just maybe, beds, okay? And have you considered it might also be to make a point about how we're treated?

So, for you, because I'm full of the milk of human kindness (no, not stored *there*), I have produced a *Rough Guide to Objectification for Dummies* – my Bitty Bobepaedia. This is a guide, not just for naïve women like me so we can spot the Bitties from miles away, but for the men for whom the only thing that figures is the figure. Bits of it.

Now, Andy was not just a Bob, he was a Dan, a Derriere

Dan, a common Bitty Bob type. The Bitty Bob range is mind-boggling but we should start with Andy, I mean Bob, I mean Dan. Because I did.

1. **Derriere Dan** aka Bottom Feeder alias Ass Man is not as ubiquitous as a Boobsy Bill (not Clinton in this instance, though he may well be one of that tribe). He may fool you more often than Boobsy Bill because unlike the latter he makes eye contact. And as their scrutiny of their preferred body part happens when you turn your back you are less aware of it. They have to be more inventive too to get the eyeful of booty they want, making them a tad more engaging. The illusion doesn't last forever though because Derriere Dan can be a pompous ass. He thinks he's revolutionary because he's bucked the trend for ogling breasts and prefers copping a feel from behind. He's convinced you'll fall over yourself to please him because he likes your burgeoning bottom when you don't. To the Dans I would say – I appreciate your sensitivity. You're on the side of all us femmes not favoured with the non-existent supermodel hips all the rage for decades (this may be changing – think Kardashian everyone). Women who aren't spring chicken anymore, 'ethnic' women with naturally bigger booties, mothers with child-bearing hips because they've, well, borne; you're our hero, Derriere Dan. But keep your distance, won't you? We'd much rather worship you from afar.
2. Then there's **Face Man**. No, no, I don't mean Dirk Benedict from The A-Team (who'd object to a bit o' bobbing with him? Not Shilpa Shetty). You'd think the Face Man was a romantic; all he wants to do is gaze at

the beauty of your face, right? But Face Man is Face Man and very pernickety about individual features. A friend told me about a guy who walks out on dates whose noses aren't centred. Just a millimetre to the left or right and he's off. And you thought *Shallow Hal* was fiction! I knew a man called Leggett with a thing for lips. Fish lips. Which worked well for me but he was prone to getting unnecessarily bitchy about the not-so-pouty, carping about the wondrous Julia Robert's 'letter-box slit' lips in the course of a conversation. 'Leg it', I'd said to him in response, or I should have. Yet the irony of the Face Man's exacting standards is that if you were to attempt to rearrange your face to fall in with his needs/society's notions of beauty/your own hankering for 'assets' you don't have, you'll only ever get censure or scorn for your pains. Especially if it's gone horribly wrong, which rom-com queen Meg Ryan found to her dismay as the rags rudely labelled her 'Old Trout Pout' after her botched lip job. Surgery, like marriage, should not be entered into lightly but if a woman chooses to have some work done to boost her self-esteem in a world that puts her down repeatedly, then why not? It's *her* body.

3. And can we forget **Hairy Scary** (he won't let us if we tried)? He doesn't mind what's behind swags of long hair as long as it's long. It's not just that most men fancy long hair on women, they appear to feel threatened by short-haired or bald women. This fear is so ingrained; it's the stuff of nightmares in fairy tales. The worst thing that happened to Rapunzel was not her kidnapping or incarceration or the blinding of her lover, but the loss of her traditionally sanctioned

long locks. In India, short-haired women deal with disapproval and disrespect more often than their long-maned counterparts. In a gallery devoted to Bollywood actresses with short-lived crops, The *Times of India* declared, 'Long hair is an asset making a girl look hot and sexier' (if I can forgive the attitude, I can't the grammar)! On top of boobs that bounce unhelpfully, wombs that immobilize once a month and bums that can't be squeezed into ... well, anything ... tight spaces, tight pants ... must we also have masses of hair obscuring our vision, tripping us up, yanked out by Baby, and the dickens to maintain? Men can go bald and be considered no less attractive (and more virile, they keep telling us. Yawn.) like Bruce Willis. Women are only women when they have wrenchable hair. As beautifully-bald-in-the-nineties Sinead O' Connor said, 'I grew too old and fat and ugly to get away with being bald.' So, the lesson to be learnt there is, if you haven't got a pretty face, cover it with a bush, a bush of hair. Actually, no, don't. Cut it short, even shear it off, sending out the powerful message that *you* decide what happens to you.

4. There are also **Leg Men** and no, it's not restricted to the beardy weirdies from ZZ Top. It's a bit of a Western import but now Asian men are just as hung up on long legs as their buddies in the west. Like hair, it seems to be the length that matters, not shape or feel or functionality (how far I can walk on my little legs doesn't appear to turn them on as much). And so, women have almost become bio-engineered to be stork-like, giving up on eating and good health, if they are not naturally predisposed to having long,

stalky legs. I won't even bother with Neck Man or **The Nibbler** or indeed, **Pussy Peep** (because which man isn't interested in our meows; that would make Bitty Bobs of all men and they're not – some of them are capable of liking more than one body part at a time). Not **Peculiar Peccadilloes Paul** though. He likes odd bits of you. It could be your big toe, the hollow behind your knees, the last knobbly bone on your spine, your belly button (a common one), your index finger, underarms, the nape of your neck or your left ear lobe. These and more are common fixations that even the average joe may have and make no bones about (but if it's your bones he digs, run; that's definitely serial-killer territory).

5. It's time to look at the most common Bitty Bob of all – Breast Man or **Boobsy Bill**! The one every woman's run into (much to Boobsy's joy) at least once. The Breast Man I got to know best was a guy I hung out with after George vamoosed. Tim was wise and well-travelled and you would never have guessed his wisdom did not extend to women. We had many wonderful conversations till one day he indulged in a touch too much wine. Soon he was telling me about the notches on his bed post – in the hundreds he said, as if I was supposed to be impressed. 'Please, please, Tim,' did he think I would say, 'make me your 347th.' I didn't, but I made the monumental mistake of forgetting that part of the conversation when we explored subjects as eclectic as Israel and the Mahabharata. He flagged down a taxi and kissed me between directions to the driver to my place. At mine, we tumbled onto the sofa and kissed some more. All

that practice had made him a nifty kisser. He tugged at my clothes but I wasn't ready. Then he tugged at my hand to lead me upstairs and I was even less ready.

'But I want to see your breasts,' he insisted.

'All in good time,' I promised.

'You're a good sized 34 D or something aren't you,' he said, peeved at what he was missing. 'No, really, I'm only a 34 B (though I was a C. C for convinced the man would have to go. And quickly).'

'Let me judge for myself. Just lift your top and jiggle them in my face like my fiancée does.' I jiggled all right. I jiggled him straight out my door. And I don't know if 'jiggle' or 'fiancée' upset me more.

But that wasn't the last of him, because this man has a million clones, with 'medical evidence' reinforcing his behaviour. The *New England Journal of Medicine* published German research which claimed a few minutes each day devoted to eyeing breasts was better for a man's health than time at the gym. 'Just ten minutes of looking at the charms of well-endowed females is equivalent to a thirty-minute aerobics work-out'. This is particularly important for men over forty who need to ogle larger breasts for better health on account of their advancing years[44]. It's all very convenient, except for us. Breasts have clearly been put on this earth, or wham-bang-centre-forward on *us* to be more precise, for men to gawp at, to grope, and to lay down the law on their exposure, use and appearance.

Remember when Angelina Jolie had her still-healthy breasts removed in 2013, because she had this teensy weensy (just 87 per cent) chance of developing breast cancer and didn't want to risk her children losing their mother? Ange said of her pre-emptive mastectomy at the time, 'I want to tell other women that my decision wasn't easy. But I'm very happy I made it. I can now tell my children they don't need to fear losing me to breast cancer. I feel empowered that I made a strong choice that in no way diminishes my femininity[45].' But did the world agree with her? The brouhaha brought boobs from inside the icky leaves of tabloids out on to the front pages of broadsheets everywhere. Suddenly, discussions about breasts were no longer restricted to the traditional locales of men's clubs and women's clinics. And the question most people seemed to be asking was – is a woman without breasts still a woman? 'People don't think so,' said Wendy Watson who had this op twenty years before Ange. 'Their biggest concern was how my husband would cope, that he would drop me because I was no longer "all woman"[46].' The world lamented the loss of Angelina's breasts because without them the woman voted the globe's sexiest time and again ceased to be sexy, or enough of a woman!

Even if we don't take the Bitty Bobs seriously, we certainly allow the media, advertising, the fashion and film industries, Mattel, as well as our mom-in-law to tell us how we should look. These entities, with their many vested interests, almost all of which have to do with making money, have decided for us women what shape and size we should be. Six feet tall, size zero and 36-24-36. And we've all bought it, though only an infinitesimally small section of us fit the above criteria. The rest of us just beat ourselves up about our shortcomings. And to show you how much about money it all is, a whole industry has sprung up around it.

From gyms to weight-loss programmes to diet foods to cosmetic surgeons, the body-shame industry is worth more than $600 billion dollars. So many of us running ourselves ragged trying to fit someone else's idea of beauty. And you can never get there because the goalpost keeps shifting. Attractiveness in women has changed over time from Rubenesque to waiflike to bootilicious once again. Some woman or the other is always being ushered out of the door because a different body shape is coming into fashion. So, no sooner than you've starved yourself into becoming anorexic and skeletal, just like they told you to, you have to feed yourself up because bottoms are back in style. You can't win.

I have been so immersed in my books and my tragedies that I haven't ever really followed fashion, changed my hair style (except when I grew my hair long for George but stood my ground on straightening it), learnt to apply make-up, bothered to diet or hit the gym. But in the last decade, I have been considered sexy. Should Kim Kardashian with her dusky skin, fish pout and Internet-breaking bottom go out of style and pale, wraithlike Kate Moss come back in, I suppose I shall have to stop thinking of myself as sexy.

But do I? Why should I? Because *Vogue* and *Cosmopolitan* say so? Well, bully for them (bullies all!). Should the shallowest end of the media (fashion magazines), the least caring of industries (cosmetics) and the most self-absorbed of people (a certain section of celebrities) be allowed to tell us what we're worth? I know women have long been wired to draw their self-worth from other's estimation of them, but if it has to be so (it shouldn't!), let it at least be from those who matter – mothers, fathers, role models.

And if we're talking worth, what's it got to do with looks? We get enough flak on almost every front without beatings with the beauty stick too. I run (on the spot, nothing heroic), I eat well enough, I do have a weakness for chocolate, balanced out by a soft spot for slinky dresses (so, from time to time, I give one up to indulge in the other). And like every other woman, all I need to do is stay within healthy bodily parameters. Every other criterion and all those people setting them, shoving them down our throats, reprimanding us for not living up to them, can go jump in the lake (a health drink lake, I suggest. Those foul, foul things).

These irresponsibly unreal expectations are making women fall ill. Twelve times more fifteen to twenty-four-year-old women die from anorexia nervosa than any other cause; older women succumb to depression as their bodies go slack; little girls in primary school watch their weight before they can even do their maths (42 per cent of all six to eight-year-old American girls want to be thinner)[47].

But men, with their dad bods, moobs and beer bellies, we are so indulgent about. They don't have to change. They definitely don't have to nearly kill themselves to achieve the right shape and look. Men's physical flaws are cute, maybe funny, but never repulsive. But this should apply to women too. And if it doesn't, it's about time we took our bodies back. Piece by precious piece. And when our bodies are ours, the standards of beauty will be ours to determine. And eventually, our lives will be a little more our own to live again.

That's what I did in those (brief, I admit) months of singledom – I set off in single-minded pursuit of the life I once had. And despite the sudden and unexpected onslaught of male interest, it had very little to do with men. It had to do with looking like myself again – cutting my hair to a clipped

Halle Berry crop, losing weight to go back to my original svelte self, dressing to please myself, which did mean my wardrobe was sexier (which worked for men too). But it was all about *me*.

I was kicking up my heels with girlfriends, doing the artsy, political things George had got in the way of. Amongst them was an interesting array of voluntary work. I began to teach English to refugees, read to underprivileged children and even write commissioned letters about (not to – though what fun that would've been!) primates in South Africa. In the process, I found myself working with a motley bunch of mavericks I hadn't thought existed in staid Sheffield. The dreadlocked Captain Five Hats who could not remember having any other name but fastidiously wore different hats for every day of the working week; the brooding, darkly-draped Goth Dawn who muttered dire predictions over her tea leaves and cake but was also a sympathetic listener; my dear friend, the madcap Carla, who fed me vegan pizza in her warm kitchen, went looking for Druid remains in the Dales with me and opened up about her own troubled past.

Life after George was gorgeous. I was able to concentrate on work, and was going places again. Literally. I was whizzing around the UK, doing the thing I did best – communicating with people through my writing, drawing and presentations, and climbing the career ladder quickly. I was mixing work and fun like any singleton would. Drinking a little, flirting a lot, throwing myself into everything and caution to the winds. Well, almost. My inner Brahmika would creep out at the most inopportune moments and stop the fun, as she had since I was a wee sprog (I did not say tree frog, I look nothing like a tree frog).

The most important thing about that short but liberating

period in my life was what I learnt about myself. One of the things I figured was that I make my best decisions when drunk. Plied with drink at an out-of-town office do the day after my divorce came through, I got tipsy for the first time in my life. The results were amazing to start with. Not a sporty type or the life and soul of a party generally, I was the only woman to volunteer to play table football with the men. I didn't just play, I whooped their sorry butts at it.

Minutes after though, my head was swimming and the floor was bucking. I could tell I wouldn't make it to my hotel room on my own. Two men – both of whom I found attractive – volunteered to help. Mark, my manager and another senior manager, Steve (although a young man, he had gone far in life, and his hungry look explained it). As addled as I was that night, something told me neither would be suitable. My eyes alighted on visiting colleague, Satish, from Coimbatore. Small, round and with brotherly blood running through his veins, he struck me as the perfect person to escort me to my room. Once there, I made a beeline for the bathroom to chuck up the contents of my mutinous stomach, while he shouted, 'Are you wokay?' through the closed door.

I awoke the next morning to sunshine, a clanger of a headache and my undergarments folded neatly on the sofa. Though, fortunately, not the ones I'd been wearing (why he folded the smalls I'd left strewn around the room while getting ready earlier in the evening remains a mystery to this day)! When I rejoined the dispersing party, Satish had already gone. There had been no embarrassment and more importantly, no nookie. My pickled brain had picked well.

Three months later, Steve and I started dating.

11

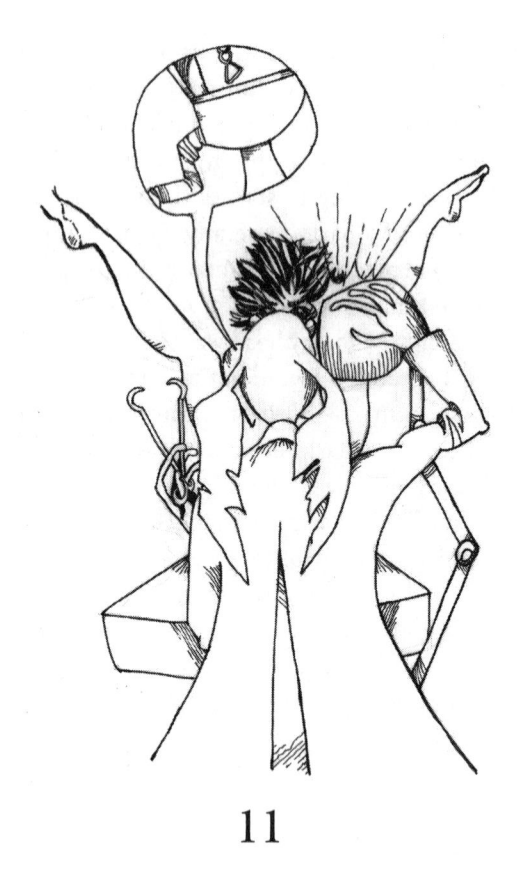

Vee for Vagina
(and Wanda, the Wilful Womb)

So far you've heard my story, but now it's her turn, her story. My vagina's. Yes, you heard me. She's figured quite largely along the way, hasn't she? But in those years when I moved from first husband to second and spawned two children, the spotlight seemed to be entirely on my vagina. And when I say spotlight, I mean literally, for most of that time I seemed to be strapped into a gynaecologist's chair with metal implements either pulling apart my womanly flaps or being inserted into the orifice between them, while a blinding light shone straight up me, warming my inner trimmings in the most uncomfortable, asexual way possible.

And yet, I've heard that this is a popular skin flick scenario, where the good doctor decides to throw away the implements and conduct the examination with his tongue. In reality, this neither happens nor would be desirable (I mean, have you seen my gynae?). Of course, other things happened to her along the way too, momentous things – soaring, sensual pleasure; terrible pain; great joy and appalling indignities (worse than the gynae's Chair of Horrors). By the time I'd dropped a child or two, suffered a hundred afterbirth problems and eased my way back to actually experiencing pleasure down there again, she – my vagina, had a full-blown personality of her own. And if post-natal tales are to be believed, she *is* full-blown, larger than life. Or if you aren't a gentleman – slack. At any rate, she has matured, become elegant if not pert anymore. An orchid rather than a dewy rose, she has many a story to tell.

Such an entity cannot, just cannot, be nameless. Yet women tend not to name their bits, like men do their willies with names like 'Willy'. What are men if not imaginative? For the more deluded, there is 'Lord of the Universe'. Men also think of and refer to their members as their pets.

'Ah,' he says sadly, 'Tiger isn't well today.' And then, as if a light bulb had come on in his head, 'Would you like to stroke him?'

'Oh, poor thing,' says she. 'Of course I will. Where's the little darling hiding?'

And out comes his little darling. Just not from under the sofa like you expected.

And we pet our privates too, don't we? Don't you sometimes find yourself running your fingers through the down, teasing strands into curls, rubbing that little button nose (all best done when alone)?

A name is obviously essential for our fluffy friend. Let's see if we can't put our finger on the perfect one:

1. Plethora: She's the gateway to so many experiences. But it sounds like something out of Asterix and she's not nearly roomy enough for a whole village of Gauls.
2. Kunti: From whom sprung so many. So appropriate but so hopelessly rude. And so likely to earn me a Hindu fatwa.
3. Vivienne. Or just Vee. This makes me think immediately of Scarlett O' Hara. Scarlet it is at that time of the month. Like her, in trouble with, and trouble for, men. And well, Vee for vagina, right?

So, I plumped for Vee because it captures the essence of my vagina in a way those pricey, pointless panty liners on the market do not. Vee, not unlike me, is adventurous but picky; a nonconformist (remains bushy when the rest of the world goes smooth), and she's lived a little but hasn't let herself go (so I'm told but The Man is biased).

You know some of her story already, of course. She was a happy little trooper, discovered fairly early by the inquisitive little girl that I was, till the early (yet again) start to bleeding, with its attendant cramps and collapses dampened her spirits somewhat. There were all those other mysterious effusions whooshing out as well. And as if these had an odour only the boys in the playground could smell (and maybe some girls –

VEE FOR VAGINA (AND WANDA, THE WILFUL WOMB) 155

certainly the one at school who insisted on stroking my arm every chance she got), they started circling her, Vee, or perhaps me, in a strange pack-like manner that was disconcerting. They would not approach though, not for years. This was India in the 1980s after all.

When the incursions began, Vee was all excited and ready, but she was to be disappointed. Years passed in which very little pleasure was to be had out of the whole inning and outing and 'oh-is-it-over-already?' business. Till the man who brought the most poking and prodding in his wake came along. Vee then became just part of the equation. As love bloomed and heartstrings entwined, she thought she would be taking a back seat, though a very pleasurable back seat – more like a sexy chaise longue – as the inning and outing for the first time did not end with 'oh-is-it-over-already?', but warm and sticky pleasure, *and* being held after.

Vee thought, ah this is the life, and that's all I'll be called upon to do from now on. But that was not to be. She became her own gateway, to much embarrassment and a lot of pain, when she allowed those tiny little eager things from the man's body into her, invading her by the millions, swimming upwards in search of the holy grail or The Womb. Once firmly ensconced there, the womb now called the shots, not Vee.

Shouldn't we name the womb too, then? Let's call her Wanda. She may not be fish-like, but the many millions who attempt to reach her shores are indeed piscine. The womb started growing a baby and became VERY, VERY IMPORTANT. Rather full of herself, you might say. But to keep Wanda and her ward healthy, Vee now underwent more poking and prodding than she thought was possible. She was no longer the VIP (Vagina Infacto Premiero) because that was Wanda now. But it was Vee who was nominated (she sure as heck didn't volunteer) as surrogate for the very public indignities pregnant women have to suffer.

And after the many insertions and examinations, Vee was finally introduced to the Joys of Childbirth. At least, she'd been told they were joys but Vee was not stupid, nuh-huh (okay, a little bit when left to her own devices). She'd experienced enough of the spread-eagling, shoving and scrutinizing already to know it wasn't going to be fun, but she had little idea of the horror awaiting her.

Childbirth Isn't Cheery

Vee was throwing up. She was disconcerted, as vaginas don't usually throw up. They leak, gush, even flood, but projectile vomiting isn't something they do. A black-green bilge called meconium cascaded out as the midwives looked on in horror and the husband was left to mop up. Meconium was the unborn baby's poo. Meconium was not just an indignity, it was trouble. The baby was not faring as well as it should.

But this was not news; we (and that would include Vee) had been rushed to hospital a week early to induce the baby, because I was in danger of developing cholestasis. Obstetric cholestasis is a serious liver ailment that can arise in pregnancy when the bile salts running from liver to gut to help digestion build up in the mother's body to an undesirable level instead, leading to stillbirths[48].

This had very little to do with Vee. In fact, she couldn't be blamed at all. But from the moment we arrived, the doctors began poking and prodding Vee something awful in their effort to induce. Then the serious pain – the contractions – began. Vee, Wanda, my tummy and legs (perfectly nice but never named), just about every inch of my body was wracked with pain. And it was unrelenting. It went on and on through that night and the next day. And the day after. In that time, they subjected Vee to a soaking (all of my pain-riven bottom half as it happens – but doesn't the bottom always get a bum deal?) in a dirty tub of hot water, which didn't help one bit.

That my husband was allowed back in the next morning to hold my hand made a huge difference to me but none at all to Vee, (man)handled by the medical staff as they kept pulling her apart and sticking things up her to check on the degree of dilation. Those metal implements will do the job, Vee winced for the hundredth time, if the pills don't.

Doc, Dopey and Bashful

Laughing gas, tremors, drugs of every sort, disorientation and an epidural later, Baby was no closer to coming into the world. But Baby needed to, because Wanda was getting fed up. Wanda was turning from snug and comforting to inhospitable. But the baby seemed to be in no hurry to arrive. And while Vee was turning desperate, and Wanda dangerous, I was blaming myself for all the complications amidst the hideous pain and anxiety.

I'd blamed myself every step of the way despite numerous reassurances that I could've done nothing about any of it. Not about the diabetes (down to race), nor the crippling SPD or Stretchy Pelvis Disorder (yes, really), the violent morning sickness that went on and on, or even Baby's defective kidney.

We'd found out at the twenty-week scan that he had a dilated left kidney. Because boys have that birth defect more often, we were informed of his sex too, though we hadn't wanted to know. A pallor of gloom had descended on us (my husband, me, even Wanda and Vee). Amidst much soul-searching about who could be responsible, my husband and I had decided to give our little boy our kidneys. Both of us. Both our kidneys. Though no known creature has ever needed four.

And now I was blaming myself for the pain that wouldn't stop, because neither Vee, who had suddenly turned bashful about opening up enough to let baby out, nor Wanda were playing ball (a baby-sized ball instead of the small, hairy ones they were used to). After thirty-three – seriously! – thirty-three hours of hard labour, the doctor finally sauntered in, stuck his nose up Vee, shook his head in disapproval and said I'd have to be cut open. And cut open I was, not a Caesarean as you might imagine, but something far more painful in the aftermath. This was an episiotomy, which involved slashing Vee's mouth to double its size so baby could be pulled out.

Vee was not happy. Wanda was relieved. And I? Despite the pain and exhaustion, I was over the moon to be holding my little bundle of ecstasy, banged up like a boxer, bruised and battered from several rounds in the ring, though he looked. That night, his eyes opened properly and he looked at me, full of wonder and admiration, as his sister did two years later, and both continue to do (on good days!). He gazed at me all night and even slashed-open Vee sighed in contentment. Wanda settled down to feeling benign about babies again, and I might have said that we all lived happily ever after, except that poor Vee did not heal for a good six months and was nearly, very nearly, operated on again.

But the very thought of more poking, prodding and pain made her heal herself overnight, so when I presented myself at the operating theatre, they took one amazed look at Vee and sent me on my way. I have always been fond of Vee, but on that day, I loved her (though it was a while before we could risk giving her any lovin').

Come to think of it, Vee had given me plenty of joy in the years leading up to the arrival of my babies. But she was a stubborn and complicated soul. She didn't like that first incursion one bit, so she held on firmly to the bit aka hymen till the oversized man's persistent thrusting allowed her to hold on no longer. Vee was desperately unhappy with the second man as well. The sorties were usually unwanted, sometimes forced, and even if it was a fine line between unsolicited and enforced, it always left Vee sore, scratched and sometimes bleeding. He didn't even have to be violent. She liked George so little that she could never get wet for him. Hence all the friction led to bruises, which led to endless soreness and the thrush. Vee didn't enjoy the George years any more than I did.

Squirming, Squirming Up the River

But Wanda I protected from George's 'squirm' (as my kids call 'em). He wanted a baby right away, to tie me down, to ensure, in his own words, that I 'didn't run away'. Befuddled though I was in every other way, I knew I didn't want to bring a baby into my uncertain, fractious life. And so my double life with George began. While he toiled away nightly (what else can I call something so without pleasure – for me as well as Vee) to get me pregnant, I popped contraceptive pills on the sly.

He found out though. He was the master of deception and I was only a novice. I hadn't hidden them away well enough. I was forced to stop taking them. And a week or so from then, when he was sure the pill no longer had any effect, he insisted on intercourse, pumping enough 'squirm' into me to ensure the sowing of his seed. The next morning, with my heart in my mouth from the possibility of a baby forming in my womb, I bought my first and last morning-after pill. I held the tiny green-and-white capsule a long time and thought about what might be inside my womb. It was unlikely there was a baby (taking into account my polycystic ovaries as well) but if there was, I believed strongly that I would do it more harm by bringing it into my squalid world than in ending its nascent little life.

Taking courage from this thought, I swallowed the magic pill. I wanted to have children but not with George. And my double life – feigned domestic harmony on the one hand, and plotting to escape to the civilized world I once knew on the other – continued apace. I was salting away money to make this escape and, after the lesson I'd learnt from hiding the pills (or not hiding them well enough), I was determined my stash wouldn't be found. I would hide it in Vee if I could. But Vee was regularly explored and no hiding place at all. Our tiny home wasn't a much better place to conceal anything and so it took as long as it did (and just a bit because I was completely out of my depth in a ha'penny pot-boiler I'd never imagined I'd find myself in). The life and death decision (my life, my maybe-baby's death) I took that day allowed me to regain control of my womb, then my body, and then my life.

Battlefield Womb

But my fight with George over Wanda was nothing new. The womb is an ancient battleground. The world has decided that a woman's womb, a body part, is more important than the living, breathing, thinking woman herself. Can you really rely on a creature that's all womb and little brain to make the correct choices for themselves and their children? Most women will put their wombs first when there is a tiny little life growing inside, but the tainted, fallen, weaker sex that we are, we can't be trusted to make the right decision. And so it's got to be a job for … no, not Superman … any man! They are all wiser and more rational. None considered more so than the Pope in the Catholic world where the power to decide what happens to a woman's body resides with him.

But Catholic Ireland is beginning to wonder if the Pope is quite as infallible as they believed (duh) after the tragic and preventable death of Indian-origin dentist Savita Halappanavar in 2012. She died from blood poisoning in the seventeenth week of her pregnancy when a timely abortion could have saved her life. Yet the fate of the 'unviable' foetus was put before that of this vital woman. Ireland is now considering a change to its abortion laws. In the meantime, a court in Northern Ireland decreed that abortions for victims of rape, incest or those with fatal foetal abnormalities should no longer be obstructed.

This was a milestone for women's rights in this deeply religious, and therefore patriarchal, part of the world from which a thousand women trek to neighbouring England, Wales or Scotland to terminate pregnancies annually. Belfast woman Sarah Ewart learnt she was carrying a fatally abnormal foetus in 2013, and would have to travel to England for a termination. Incensed, she invited the BBC to film her story, which led to such a furore in Northern Ireland that it brought them closer to changing the law finally[49]. It's not a done deal, yet it's a better deal than given to many, even most, women around the world. Most will continue to have little say in what happens to their bodies, and their lives, once impregnated.

In 'liberal' America, the pro-life/pro-choice war rages on and it's a real battle where abortion clinics are firebombed and people die because their opponents are 'pro-life'. Eleven people have been murdered by anti-abortionists in the US since 1993; over 200 clinics have been bombed or set on fire since the late seventies[50]. Of course, women die all the time from abortions. As abortion is either prohibited or severely limited to a quarter of the world, dodgy clinics and dubious doctors thrive. And they kill. More than half the abortions carried out in less prosperous parts of the world are unsafe. As a result, 70,000 women die from them every year. Another 2 to 7 million women survive the butchery but become damaged or diseased.

A baby's life is precious, any mother will agree, long before it comes into the world. I sang to my babies when they were 'little beans' in my tummy as if they were already fully conscious, full-fledged children. And while I have never had an abortion (though the conservative would fervently argue that the morning-after pill is the same thing), I do believe that as long as it is early enough to be safe and not a procedure repeatedly resorted to in place of contraception, there can be very valid reasons for a woman to terminate her pregnancy. If her life is at risk, if she's been forcibly impregnated, or barely a child herself, the need for one shouldn't even be questioned. Bringing a baby into an abusive home can be worse too for both mother and baby than choosing to end the pregnancy safely and early. Each case is different and blanket bans clearly do more harm than good. Instead, we should provide young women *and* men with the open and honest education that will equip them to make the right decisions.

So while I was saddened to have to take action at all, I grieved much less than years later when Wanda misplaced another little soul. But then, to her credit, she had brought two beautiful babies safely into my world in the meantime. And because, after the horror of childbirth the first time, I had chickened out of doing it the 'natural' way and gone for a Caesarean the next, Vee had been a happy bunny through it too. Vee of course had been a contented coot (of the Avian variety and nothing at all to do with nits – yikes) for a while because a man had finally been found who could make her happy but it took a few tries for even that man to figure her out.

VEE FOR VAGINA (AND WANDA, THE WILFUL WOMB) 163

Vee, you see, was no less complicated than me. Almost courtly in the very early stages of our relationship, it was only when we first attempted penetrative sex (oh, but we'd had fun enough leading up to it), that we discovered it couldn't be done. We had engaged in the usual foreplay on the sofa. After a gorgeous dinner, putting aside hot cups of coffee, we got steamier still. Kissing, stroking, and fondling, we found our way up the stairs and on to my bed. I wrapped myself around him, easing him in as he began thrusting, both of us grinning beatifically all the while. But then he stopped. Stopped and looked aghast. He couldn't find his way in. We changed positions. And pace. Rushing it in as if to catch Vee unawares, or sliding in ever so slowly in case he had missed the opening in his haste earlier. Then we tried lubrication. Tongue, gel, strawberry jam later, we were no closer to getting ... well, closer. Embarrassed and confused, we gave it up for the night, curling into each other and sleeping (or pretend-sleeping while worrying about whose fault that had been).

A couple of weeks later, we were more in love, and farther away from managing any actual intercourse. Every attempt started out beautifully, but perished at the penetrative stage. Even a sexy four-poster bed in a pretty, rose-smothered cottage in picturesque Ross-on-Wye hadn't opened Sesame (Vee is my vagina. Sesame, the caverns within, of course). Try as he might, muh man just could not get in. He was hard enough. I was undeniably ready. It was as if I was still a virgin, though I'd been put through a rigorous course of penetrative sex for the whole five years before that. It confounded and distressed us. Our relationship, the first really happy one I'd been in, felt destined to stay unconsummated and therefore, appeared doomed. Because whoever heard of paramours who didn't, no, couldn't *ram*? We then, both of us individually and ever-so-secretly, snuck off to doctors. Vee wasn't happy. She'd not minded being left alone for a few months. Quite the opposite. But there she was again, lying on a doctor's couch, upended and inelegantly lit, while the doctor, fortunately female, so more likely to sympathize with whatever was the matter (I didn't know what Vee, or more importantly my guy, thought it might be, but I dreaded being told it was a freak case of a reformed hymen or worse, The Big C), rummaged around inside me. And then with a big grin declared, 'You have a u-bend.'

'A what?' I said.

'You know, like a toilet,' she said.

Oh fab, I thought, what a wonderfully romantic thing to have to explain to your new lover: 'My vagina has a u-bend like a toilet which means the pipe is kinda loopy (like its owner).'

'But I've had perfectly normal sex before,' I said to the cheerfully grinning doc.

'Is this a new partner?' she asked, continuing to look pleased with herself as my heart sank at the thought that she would just dismiss us as mismatched – u-bended and noo-bended – and that would be that.

As it turned out, women can have loopy pussies and men wonky cocks, sometimes these work well together and you never even realize there are kinks to them. But along comes the love of your life and the angle his dick's at doesn't make the most natural fit for your foof. Or at least, not at first. But a little bit of practice and experimentation would fix that, the good doctor said, and we got to it right away. And strangely (or not so strangely; all in the mind as it really is), as soon as we knew that it wasn't going to be a problem, it stopped being one.

One wonderful winter's day, in a snowed-in log cabin in

Derbyshire where we'd holed up for Christmas, he flung my pretty pink bra and pants to the heavens and slipped in as if there had never been a hitch. And he was such a perfect fit, so firm and snug inside, that another first happened. At the grand old age of thirty and with a lover or two behind me, I came for the first time. I climaxed with him in a warm gush and with a happy scream. The rest of that particular holiday was devoted to little else. And while the snow storm raged outside for a week making many a grouch across England very grumpy, we stayed in bed and made Vee very, very happy.

12

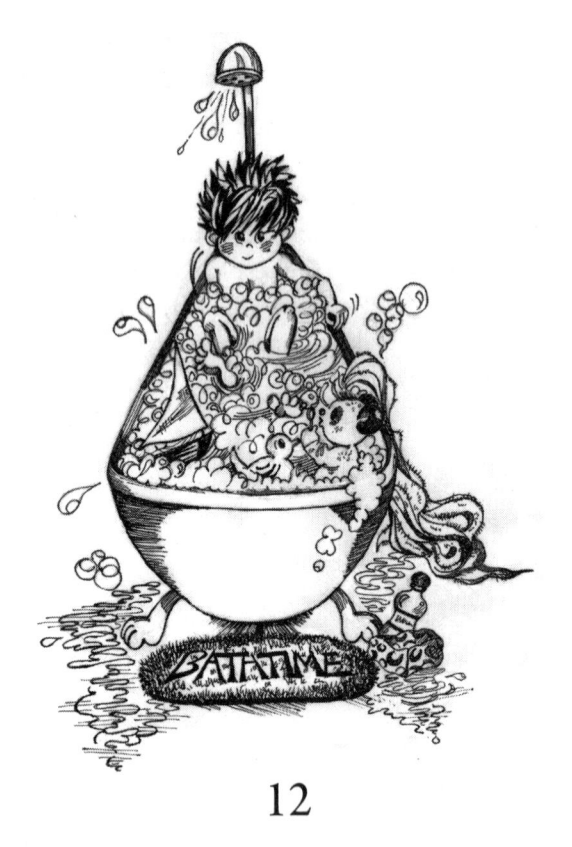

Nudity Begins at Home

Having found the man I wanted to spend my life with, and having had his offspring, I settled down to being a mother. No, settle is not something I do. I took a sabbatical from 'work' to bring my babies up right. Or as-near-as-dammit. I had issues with my own upbringing and wanted to turn it all on its head for my children. The plan was not to be just any old mother.

Oh no, I was going to be a pretty rad mother. Certainly rad if not pretty (how *do* you do pretty with poop in your hair and puke down your front?).

I decided to forego the usual reading of billions of blue, blistering baby books before their birth, one or two Lamaze classes I did attend but that was enough, nor did I have a cutesy-flutesy baby shower or allow any old wives' tales about child-rearing to be shoved down my thickening throat. I was going to do it my way. Despite crashing and burning repeatedly, I still wanted to be individual, and that usually meant going about things as differently as possible from how it had been done before, especially by my family. That meant flouting Indian conventions, shouting down my inner wimp and throwing inhibitions to the winds.

Throwing things to the winds was easy in the forest where we lived. I had placed myself far enough away from conventions of any kind, certainly those I grew up with, to make it possible to live the life I wanted with my little family. After my bruised boxer baby, we had a tiny, slim-limbed little girl whose hair stood on end as if in fright when she first came into the world. Both blossomed beautifully once safely home in our sunset-red brick house in Sherwood Forest. And that had as much to do with the sylvan setting we'd found for their early years, as it did with our accommodating approach to parenting – something I shall explain in a bit.

From the window of their lulling lavender nursery, was a view that saw apple orchards, reed-filled ponds, a tree house put up by some young scallywags, and a magical wall. A thousand-year-old wall of sturdy stone that belonged to the manor house beyond the orchards, which had sheltered duelling Byrons and dancing bears in its time. But it was a silent house now with only the chimney tops visible, and the occasional gardener we espied through the apple trees. Our own home was like Baby Bear's bed, neither too big nor too small but just right. A solid seventies house with sunny rooms, so shielded from civilization, that we could barely hear the hum of cars. What we were surrounded by instead were birds, squirrels and even foxes who vied to outdo each other in noise and colour. But little could match my toddlers' decibel levels when excited, or the blur of rainbow hues and lightning-quick darts that they became at play.

I had no chance of keeping up, so I took my laptop to our creaky Victorian swing and attempted to write instead. Did I mention the swing was a chipped green merging beautifully with the stand of trees behind? When we first moved in, even the house was green. From the front door to our bedroom, it was all a dark green. We had to paint over the last with an iridescent ivory, or no babies would have been made in its eerie gloaming. So, there was good and bad in our forest home, till we made it our own. As we did the upbringing of our children. A vital part of that education was about the human body, sex, and sexual rights.

Living without interfering mausis, peeping toms or 'concerned' neighbours (the last two being the same), gave us the freedom to grow our children our way, alongside tomatoes, beans, cucumber, chillies and more, all of which went into big simmering pots in the evenings (the veggies, not the kids)! But the children did flourish like our garden. They grew fast, and we were as guilty as other parents of complaining about that even as it pleased us no end to watch them shoot like beanpoles towards the sun. They also grew into well-rounded personalities like the juicy squashes in the gold-green chequered patch near the wall.

Bollywood, Hollywood

Most of my generation grew up loved too, but how many of us became well-adjusted adults, aware of and at ease in the world? Especially the world beneath our navels? Let me count them on my fingers. Gosh, that didn't take long, did it? We grew up awkward half-people because of the ignorance into which we were deliberately waylaid. Boys and girls alike were equally unaware of what the tiddly bits beneath their tummies were for. The very mention of sex was usually accompanied by heavy sweating, with feeble attempts to conceal it with frightened titters.

As for homosexuals, transgender people and the like, they were the bogeymen of our childhood, freaks with whom the slightest contact could blight our lives forever. Regardless of whether every parent was as guilty of misrepresenting or suppressing the facts, we grew up as gauche as the generations before us. Oh, they meant well (they were 'protecting' us from the scary stuff like, er, our own bodies), and some could even be described as liberal (they let you watch Mary Poppins kiss Dick – Dick Van Dyke), but we all still got the wrong messages about sex and the human body. Since they mostly kept mum about it, Hollywood, Bollywood, *Mills and Boons* and the weird uncle who liked sitting you on his knee filled in the gaps.

Hollywood taught us that sexual freedom was in how many we made out with rather than the choices we made (Hollywood itself, therefore, became a choice that was taken away from us unless old, grainy and sterilized). And many of the 'lessons' out there were, not surprisingly, for girls. Because we have always needed to be told our place.

Bollywood impressed upon us growing girls the importance of unquestioningly toeing the (sexual) line set down by the man in our life, be it father, husband or some dirty old man that's made it his business. Or we might as well be dead. And often were, mid-way through the movie. *Mills and Boon* taught us that sex is best when forced upon us, usually by a nasty boss or Arab Sheik with a harem habit. And the less said about the things your 'uncle' told you as you perched uncomfortably on his knee, the better. Then there was the stuff we picked up in the playground, and I don't mean the odd half-chewed candy (less likely to upset young tummies than the whispered stories). We were told bizarre tales from the bedroom, which the teller only half-understood herself. I was wary of boys' fingers for ages, because I was warned that that's how they slipped babies in. I know better now (such a relief, as I do so enjoy them). But credulous little ones are still being told preposterous tales, 'Touching your pee-pee will make it fall off', or 'Kissing gives you AIDS.'

If you can pooh-pooh playground patter, there's plenty else out there that's harder to discredit, especially when it's in the omniscient, irreproachable media. 'Men, I know you think your woman isn't the type who wants to be taken. But trust me, she is. Every girl wants to get her hair pulled once in a while. If your wife says "no", turn her around and rip her clothes off. She wants to be dominated.' This is from a book called *Love Italian Style* by reality TV star Melissa Gorga[51]. Little league compared to the ridiculously successful, mind-numbingly awful *Fifty Shades of Grey*, the doormat's guide to delirious domination by a freak. With bilge like that taken to the bosoms of many a mom (and dad!), and the impact on our children of the skewed subliminal sex messages in video games, for example, how can we even expect our young ones to grow up to understand and enjoy their bodies in a happy, uninhibited yet realistic way? And their sexual rights too, whether child, woman or homosexual?

By not leaving the 'educating' to others, that's how. Because guess what happens when we pass the buck? 300,000 American women are raped every year. One in twenty British women is a victim of at least one serious sexual assault. 66 per cent of Turkish police officers believe that 'the physical appearance and behaviours of women tempt men to rape'. 74 per cent of women in Mali say their husband has the right to beat them if they withhold sex. And, in India, there's Nirbhaya. Not one but hundreds of thousands.

Let's Talk About Sex, Babies

My children have the benefit of what most of my generation (and those before us) didn't: a parent who talks (endlessly) about sex. But even if you don't enjoy it nearly as much as I do (the talking ... okay, not just the talking), you can still do your damnedest to explain it well. Not by pussyfooting around the really important bits. Yes, pussy. Tell them about that too. So, they'll titter while they learn. Where's the harm? Knowing too much is better than too little. It arms them against assault, disease, heartache, and transgressions of their own. And it is undeniably better than the gaping vacuum with the occasional bizarre bit of misinformation rattling around that was our sex education.

Their dad and I wanted to hide nothing from the kids. Or as little as possible. We wanted them to grasp (metaphorically and literally) the human body. See it for the lovely but commonplace thing that it is, thereby demystifying and destigmatizing it all at once. If it isn't shrouded in mystery, it can neither be beast nor bait. It's like toast for breakfast (still scrumptious with chocolate or cheese) but not any more mysterious, obfuscated or unnaturally alluring. We did not, of course, set up a naturist commune or spend all day in the nude! We just decided not to turn prudes and hide our light under bushels (or jiggly bits in unnecessary layers). And because I think it's worked rather well, let me share with you my six piddles of wisdom (pillars you say? If you've got kids, piddles it is).

1. Why not wear what you would have worn round the house before the children came along? If that's not full body armour, then it shouldn't be with kids around either. Kids have a lot of questions and you might have to explain your sartorial choice of shorts over, say, a salwar ('which Leena's mommy wears'). But tell them why that is and then carry on; you have to be yourself and not Mother Hubbard.
2. You may not want to lock the door in their faces when you're changing (wouldn't you much rather know they are safe than saintly?). And you know what? They aren't saintly, they never were. They, like you, came into this world with questions and thoughts about their bodies. And the urge to explore. Of which they've done plenty already. Trust me.
3. To see you at ease in your skin will give them immense confidence in their bodies, and this will act like an invisible shield against unreal media and social expectations. Your free-spirited children will blossom into self-respecting adults.
4. Don't stop their explorations of their own bodies. It's normal, healthy and a much better way to learn about the human body than many others out there, which you might just drive them to if you don't allow this simple pleasure. Do flip back to chapter 1 if in doubt.
5. Maybe have baths with them when they're little? It

gets them used to the human body. If they grab, ease the slightly inappropriate extremity out of their grip and replace it with a bath toy. It's all squidgy to them.
6. Try to answer all their questions, all the time, especially the ones about sex. This one is quite often the hardest to do, but also the most important. Mine, at three and four, had a preschool version of the birds, bees, tiddlers, 'front-bottoms' and what they instinctively refer to as 'the nibbles' talk.

Shall we do a little quiz now to see if I've managed to turn you into an airy-fairy-the-body's-not-scary hippie chick like me?

1. If your child were to see you in the buff, should you:
   a) Scream, hide or scold to cover your embarrassment.
   b) Insist you are, in fact, wearing clothes, like the befuddled emperor.
   c) Act like nothing untoward has happened, because nothing has.
2. If they were to ask a particularly knotty question about sex, how would you answer it? Like our son innocently piped up one day, 'Daddy, what is bondage?'
   a) Send him to his room (because you're pretty sure there's no bondage equipment there and by the time he's allowed back out, he might have forgotten).
   b) Waffle on about Somerset Maugham's novel, *Of Human Bondage*, hoping you can bore them into losing interest.
   c) Explain enough to quell their curiosity so they don't go looking for the answer elsewhere, but not so much as to scare them (hey, it's a pretty scary subject, even for you perhaps, so I get that you'd want to keep it brief, but don't ignore the question. They'll only google it, and guess what they'll find).

Analysis: If you picked 'c' twice and emphatically, congratulations! You're well on your way to HippieChickhood!

Of course, this openness can and does lead to embarrassing situations. At a recent extended family dinner, our little girl loudly informed everyone that her parents had been 'bobbing up and down on each other AGAIN!' In fact, it was a fully clothed cuddle, the mildest of PDL moments (public displays of love because calling it affection doesn't cut the custard). Would it matter though if they had happened on more? I would rather have my kids think of sex as wholesome, maybe even mundane and obviously, totally for the doddering, than something filthy, furtive and fly-by-night. Because when something is forbidden, it follows that it has to be taken by force. British sociologist Stevi Jackson explains how the home is the first place where children weigh up what's right and what's wrong. But their need to know is often thwarted by evasion and the sexual repression of their parents. 'In attempting to protect children from sex, we expose them to danger,' she argues. 'In trying to preserve their innocence, we expose them to guilt. In keeping both sexes asexual and then training them to become sexual in different ways, we perpetuate sexual inequality, exploitation and oppression.'[52]

But parents and schools have been traditionally wary of teaching their children about the birds and the bees. This toughest of jobs, the most important of jobs, is left to the banal media and the profiteering sex industry. Every year from 2013, Channel 4 has run a *Real Sex* season to help Britain regain 'a healthy perspective on sex, in a world where pornography, fantasy and fetish are considered the norm by many[53].' But with shows like *Sex Box* that set couples canoodling in a box, a concept that's hardly out of the box, they were never going to usher in a sex education revolution. Plus, what could you possibly learn about sex and the human form when you don't even know which part is jammed against your face? Yet this coitus cardboardus did get people talking, and if one or two of these conversations were parent-child chats where sexual fears, misconceptions and expectations were addressed, then it was well worth the trite TV.

As for the porn industry, I'm fairly 'c'est la vie' about it too. Where there's a demand, there'll be a supply, but let this demand be an exclusively adult one. Because children and adolescents exposed to the norms of this industry are indelibly affected. What do they learn from watching films that often pander to the darkest of male desires? They learn that women are objects to be 'taken'. Boys are led to believe that girls who say 'no' really mean 'yes'. Girls are told they should shut up and take it. The message that is clearly being sent out is that women are not worthy of respect.

No young person exposed to this unequal, unreal sex could possibly learn how happy, warm and giving it can be between ordinary people. It is a well-documented fact that even adults find real-life sex difficult to deal with once they are hooked on porn. So, do talk about everyday sex with your babies. Or if you're bashful, you could look for a good, age-appropriate, educational video (screwing up your courage to answer questions afterwards!). Campaigning, like a group of parents I know, for their school to start a relevant and effective sex education programme is a great idea too. Please don't leave it to someone else.

Badass Mashima

Trips back to the motherland only strengthens this conviction that parents need to take the matter by the scruff of the neck. The prevalence of sex-related crimes in India suggest that women are seen as bait as well as trophy in a sexual game. And the archaic and misogynistic pronouncements from Bollywood, politicians and the media, to name but a few culprits, only serve to reinforce this impression for far too many men. Revolutions, however, usually start small and often in the home, so it really is up to the babas, ammas, chaachas and mashimas to sort out khoka/beta.

Just how much it's needed became apparent at South City Mall in Kolkata on a busy Sunday a couple of years ago. While mooching about happily by myself, I realized that I, no less a 'mashima' than the next one (by virtue of having crossed forty), and worthy of our time-honoured tradition of Mother Worship, was being tailed by a pack of ridiculously young men. I could see my snug jeans had shorted their rudimentary thought circuit, causing confusion. As that famous Kalki Koechlin anti-rape video said, it was my fault. So I decided to fix it, by reminding that brazen bunch what it is a mashima is made of (*not* sugar and spice and all that's nice).

I stopped and turned to glare at them. They sneered and kept advancing. But instead of the little woman scuttling away as they had expected, I stood my ground and began to loudly tell people around me what dolts those boys were and what they'd been up to. People tittered. A few came up to ask me what was going on. And then I saw *them* creeping away, red-faced they'd been seen off by a woman. Never underestimate a mashima. Or any woman, of any age, who knows what a mashima knows! I felt like shouting at their retreating backs. Predatory men, prowling solo or in packs, are no match for a badass bitch. Men like that, fed on the media tosh and porn twaddle of women as weak and subservient, back off when women defy them. Not only do we women need to remember that, but remind men of it as often as we can too.

Boys Will Be Boys

So, sexual frankness is next to godliness and nudity begins at home (or something like that). But another life lesson was needed to round off this particular part of my kids' education. It was key to their becoming the adults we wanted them to be. It was about R.E.S.P.E.C.T (sing it with me).

Boisterous little boys, all flying limbs and curiosity, are lovely and innocent and mean absolutely no harm when they come crashing into you, but unless you teach them well, they grow up to be men who continue to do the same, and that's not lovely at all. Hence, boys need to learn to respect other people's bodies, physical space and the right to sexual choices, whether they are in line with what they themselves want or not.

That doesn't mean girls don't need to learn the same. But girls don't manhandle bodies, violate physical space and impose their own sexual choices on others as often. Yes, yes, there was the incongruous, and rather terrible if true, story of a group of college girls in Delhi who were luring autorickshaw drivers to their rooms to have their wicked way with them. After which they would keep the man's driver's licence as a trophy. The police found a tottering pile of these documents in the girls' rooms when the traumatized drivers complained.

Hang on a minute. Luring autorickshaw drivers to their rooms to assuage their sexual needs? Really? Wouldn't virginal boys from their college have been the more likely victims of the boundless lust of these women? And those IDs the police found so conveniently stashed in the girls' rooms incontrovertibly proving their guilt … a bit too convenient? Sounds like a 'philmi phrem up' to me, but then maybe I'm being a reverse sexist here. Yet all the Pirito Poti organizations in the world can't convince me that it's not our little boys we need to teach a tad more sensitivity to when it comes to sexual rights.

And so we did, but we taught them both. We taught our children to respect differences, whether it was in body parts or sexual choices. The body parts bit was easy because they had such an innate curiosity about it. Talk of private parts and giggled rhymes about unlikely people 'sitting in a tree, K-I-S-S-I-N-G', chanted at home or shouted out loud on the tram into town, with everyone twisting round to listen, were very much a part of our everyday lives.

Sitting in our sun-dappled garden one beautiful summer's day, listening to Ella warble *'Summertime and the livin' is easy'* with the children playing nearby, I was reminded how important this lesson of respect for the sexual rights of others is, when I suddenly heard from over the fence a child jeering an age-old rhyme to another. 'What are little boys made of? Frogs and snails and puppy dogs' tails.'

That boys are born dirty, nasty, and violent is not just a slight from a nursery rhyme that children hurl at each other; it's also a belief as old as time, and perpetuated constantly in the modern world. 'Boys will be boys' and cannot be expected to rise above their primitive DNA, we are told, ad nauseam. If we are to believe Indian politician Mulayam Singh Yadav, being a boy involves occasionally, mistakenly, committing rape and horrific sexual violence[54].

And this isn't just 'Third-World' thinking. Following a US government probe into Montana's handling of rape cases, it was found that they routinely shelved legitimate ones. Or humiliated victims even as they half-heartedly prosecuted the perpetrators. Rape, they clearly believed (like far too many others), was just men letting off manly steam after some vile woman had led them astray. So, no surprise then when the mother of a five-year-old questioned the Montana county attorney on the negligible punishment her daughter's attacker had received that he said – you guessed it – 'Boys will be boys[55].'

These blithe generalizations suggesting that boys are nasty by nature hurt boys as much as girls. Even as we tell them that's who they are and we expect nothing more, after every rape, acid attack and murder, we spend interminable television hours and miles of column space castigating them for their inability to keep their tackle in their pants and their inner animal in check. But it's us – mothers, fathers, teachers, leaders and the media, who continue to create such men.

There's an apocryphal story about Isaac Newton where his father, disappointed at the amount of time Isaac spent looking at the world, exhorted him to 'be a man', setting him the task of chopping down a tree. Isaac decided to sit under it and dream instead. Then down came an apple, and gravity was deciphered, changing our world forever. Had he done the 'manly' thing of chopping the tree, what, other than taking a life, would he have achieved?

Our little boy will not be sent out to chop down trees (only conventions). We have a deep-thinking seven-year-old boy. He isn't keen on kicking a ball around with heftier classmates, but he runs, jumps, and hollers with the best of them. He also likes to write stories, build robots and pick out my clothes for a party. Should I, in horror, send him to football camp, boxing classes or down to the pub to let some of that blustering aggression rub off on him? No, I think I will let him read in his beloved patch of green beneath the walnut trees, run like the wind through the forest, and build his robots in the quiet of his sky-blue bedroom. And take an interest in clothes when he wants to.

I have a multitalented daughter who likes to kick a ball but is equally adept at dancing. She has a horror of pink (pressed as it is upon little girls as the only shade they should like), but is a dab hand with colours and draws like a dream. She will race to the finish before everyone else with the maths and sciences as much as languages at school, but won't hesitate to stop and help a friend if they were falling behind.

The Rainbow Connection

They are both shaping up to be fine, multifaceted folk, unconcerned by gender stereotypes and respectful of individual differences, including those of sexual orientation. This feels especially important at a time when the bigoted seem to be working extra hard to turn the clock back to the Dark Ages. The Russian government prohibited the 'propaganda of non-traditional sexual relations' in 2013, with subsequent veiled threats from Putin of a pogrom against Russian homosexuals and a concomitant rise in harassment[56].

Not to be left behind, at the fag end of 2013, the Indian Supreme Court recriminalized homosexuality. Within a year 600 people had been arrested for 'carnal intercourse against the order of nature'[57]. In many Middle Eastern states, you can still be executed for it. It is also illegal to be gay in thirty-six out of fifty-four African nations. You could be jailed for life just for articulating desire, as Cameroonian Roger Mbede found out[58]. In the West, you won't be executed, imprisoned or face as much disapproval at home for being gay. Not these days. But there are enough instances of discrimination, bullying and random jackbooted attacks to suggest homophobia is alive and well.

The concept of oppressing people for their sexual orientation is so archaic, it boggles the post-Palaeolithic mind. Ironically, while it's ridiculously old fashioned to be anti-gay, being gay is a very old fashion indeed; there's plenty of proof it's always existed in humans, with depictions on ancient Hindu temples and references in early Greek and Egyptian texts just the tip of the iceberg. It flourishes in the natural world too, in 1,500 animal species[59]. Here in the woods, our babes have seen relatives in happy relationships with same-sex partners. To them, it's as natural as Daddy and Mommy being together. Coming home shaken when a schoolmate insisted 'girls can't marry girls', they asked if that could be true.

Sitting them down with bickies and milk in our large, warm kitchen, I reminded them of Aunties Lisa and Jane. I told them how happy Lisa and Jane were after a decade together. How completely at ease in a world that only half-accepted them. How keen to live a good life and do the right thing by society. And though the wintry wind lashed mercilessly at our kitchen window, my children glowed with pleasure at the thought of their loving, lesbian aunts. 'I remember when Aunties Lisa and Jane got married,' our son beamed. 'What a wonderful day that was!' my little girl finished for him.

I will never change the world. But together, my husband and I strive to be a really cool Free-spirited Momma and a wickid, wickid (in the street sense of the word) Warlock Dad. We will have a little révolution in our own home, where the things the last generation did and didn't do – from the condemnation of masturbation to keeping mum about the birds and the bees – are completely overturned and re-engineered.

And if the kids were to tell other children and our reformation extend down the street, we would have changed our world for the better after all. They might even want to pass on this *totally original* slogan I coined: Liberté, égalité, fraternité.

Liberty: Let's give our children the freedom to love their bodies and its urges.

Equality: How about we teach boys and girls to respect their differences and acknowledge the similarities?

Fraternity: Let's not forget that we are all 'queer', some more than others, and it's not just about sexuality.

As our children grow up as beautiful inside as out (to this mother's eyes anyway) as Sherwood in its summer glory, as nicely rounded as the ruby-red apples in the orchard beyond our walls, and as sensitive as the delicate indigo flowers that spring from the roots of our thousand-year-old trees, we can be justifiably happy in having been the parents we meant to be. But in teaching them about love, sex and the beauty of the body, did we forget something for ourselves along the way?
Mo' jiggy wit it.

13

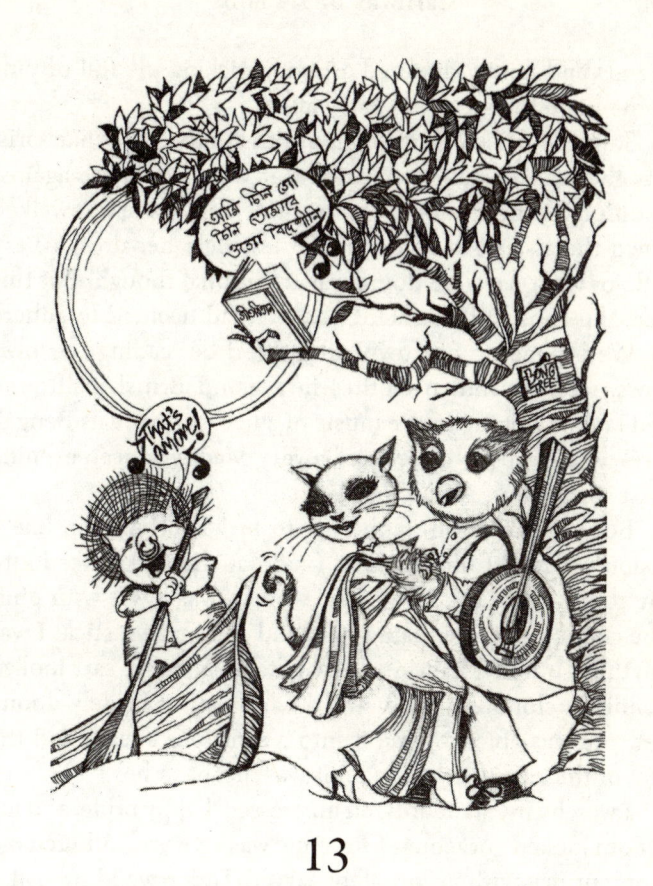

Sex After Marriage aka SAM I AM

My sari was unravelling. My sumptuous six yards of deep onion-pink silk was refusing to stay on and I, like any bride, was getting anxious. In fact, I felt like a cross between Alice's White Rabbit (I'm late, I'm late, for a very important date) and Eliza Doolittle's dad (Get me to the church on time!) as friends and family fluttered around, sticking me full of pins in the hope the sari would stay afloat.

Steve, who usually helped me with knotty things like saris, was the man I was marrying, and it would be quite against tradition for the groom to see the bride before she was walked down the aisle to his side (much less help her dress). Very little of what we were doing was traditional though. But this one, this most inconvenient one, we had decided to adhere to. We'd made up our own rules. We'd be reading our own vows, wearing Indian clothes in a grand British ballroom, and later, swinging to the music of a live jazz band as Bengali terracotta lamps twinkled and a very Mediterranean evening feast was had.

But the sari wasn't adhering to *me*! Drat! When, like a vision, a friend from Madurai (via Manchester) walked into the room and I was saved. The woman was a wiz with pins. She could pin an elephant to a cloud and make it stick. I was anything but elephantine at that stage, but that sari looked definitely cloudlike, puffy and a harbinger of bridely doom. Yet, she was able to tame it into a sensuous sheath and the rest of the day was the dream it was meant to be.

I was, by my standards, an unstressed, happy bride, and my groom looked gorgeous. The venue was an ivy-smothered old stone priory with an ornately carved Tudor wedding hall – splendid. The lawns of the priory, where we had champagne and canapes before lunch, were the lushest green, strewn with guests, flowers and baby rabbits (a hint from ever-impatient Mother Nature surely).

But the finest thing about that day was that my family could attend this wedding, unlike my previous one, which had been hurriedly conducted on a dreary day in Sheffield in a government office with a one-armed registrar presiding over it (the best bit!).

Yet, nothing, not even the most joyous of wedding days, can be flawless, and so set in a long power cut, in a country that nearly never had any. A nod to my origins in Kolkata, I decided, where 'load-shedding' occurred daily. It ended just as we'd begun to worry about the food waiting to be cooked and the guests going hungry.

I was disabused of the notion that we'd got our guests sustenance in time when, after desserts were done and coffee quaffed, a whisper drifted to me from a nearby table.

'Just one more,' said the man pleadingly.

'NO! You are a disgrace, what if anyone should see you?' a woman barked back.

I smiled to myself. Was a very drunk member of our party getting his knuckles rapped by his more sober partner? Then I heard her hiss, 'Put that meat back on the table,' and turned to see Uncle Winston, wizened and rather furtive-looking (and now I knew why), stuffing his pockets with the beautifully braised pork chops we'd served as one of our mains. I had no idea how he'd amassed so many (had he asked for extras/gathered everyone's leftovers/managed a quick run to the kitchen for more?).

I quickly looked away, catching the tail of his whine, 'What if dinner's late too?' Dinner wasn't late. But dinner, on top of a delayed but humongous lunch, followed by drinking, dancing and non-stop nattering with our guests, meant we were so bushed by bedtime, that my groom and I managed to do nothing sensible with my prettily pruned bush that night. Poor Vee. We staggered to our flower-strewn nuptial bed to fall upon it and sleep like the dead.

It wasn't till a week later, as we wound our way up a green hillside in Corfu in a tin-can of a hired car, that we felt those familiar flip-flops in our tummy that told us, not that we'd smuggled some priory bunnies out in our clothes, but that we were finally rejuvenated enough to be in the mood for lurve. With sparkling blue seas all around us and the green of the olive groves a calming jade, this was the kind of place that lulled your senses, sharpening only those which were usually ignored in the humdrum course of the day. So, although we picked up the scent of oranges wafting across from the neighbouring orangery, wondered at the twinkling stars that appeared to dot the grass at dawn, only to find they were glow-worms grazing, and felt the warm glow of the sun at mid-day as we lay by our tranquil pool-for-the-week, these were gentle sensations compared to the ravenous hunger that would overtake us every few hours and send us running to the pantopoleío for fresh fish to grill with pungent feta and ripe tomatoes.

And if the pangs of hunger were strong, the urge to tangle was even more so. Not only at night between the crisp sheets of our cavernous bed, but in the mornings, waking to find those sheets flung off and our bodies glowing pearly in the timorous dawn light flooding our room, we would wade into each other as if after a long drought. Yet while coochie-cooing in our own cabana was quite the done thing, we were struck by the urge to fandango in the most unlikely places.

'Ooh look at that olive grove,' said my new husband, stopping the car to gaze longingly at what looked like a very large garden-waste heap of twigs and moss and leaves.

'That an olive grove?' I shot back, peering over his shoulder, 'it looks like compost to me.' And I sniffed the air disdainfully, to indicate it smelt like it too.

'Shall we?' said the husband, entwining his fingers with mine and giving my hand a little tug.

'Yes, let's!' I replied, looking into his eyes and seeing (and smelling) nothing else besides.

Such fecundity, both Corfu's and ours, could only lead to one thing. And it wasn't long after our return from that abundant island that we found ourselves in the family way, with more to follow less than two years later.

And so we learnt another life lesson of almost as much importance soon after; that the beautiful, maddening, taking-up-all-our-time-and-then-some product of our mating would ensure the latter became a very rare pleasure. As rare as sleep and *almost* as longed for. Pregnancy is the first nail in the coffin of getting nailed. Sleep dies a death too. There's barely a position that's comfortable by your second trimester because your stomach is like a sack of coal you've insisted on lugging around with you (and into bed too). There are hard bits and lumpy bits, because Baby's discovered weak points she can drill through with her toes to make her escape. But if you can't sleep, you can't stay up and make whoopee with your partner either, because the last thing you want on top of the (sometimes very large) extrusions, are smaller (um, yeah, much) intrusions.

Oh, there are phases in your pregnancy when you're as horny as an off-key bugle (in need of a rub and a blow), but the minute you act on it, desire disappears as discomfort takes over. Sex stays off the roster even after the kids arrive. By the time your little monsters/marvels/munchkins have hit toddlerhood, opportunities do arise, but you just want to … zzzz … huh, what, where were we? The libido recovers (ever so) slowly. And runaway sex comes home.

Yet, now it requires scheduling, strategic thinking, minute planning, precision engineering and ruthless execution. The rewards, we know, are enormous (without that big baby bump in the way, intrusions feel larger too). But between thinking it a good idea to schedule sex that month and actually lying back having your breasts licked while your fingers grasp your partner's shaft (very, very tightly, after all, who's responsible for everything you've been through?) is a long tortuous road like no singleton can imagine. Or maybe they can, which is why they stayed single!

Single Dating Vs Married Mating

Many of my single friends are very Zen; they may be pushing forty but they can't be bothered to scavenge (look for likely people left over from the great rush to bag a partner in our twenties and thirties). If they do, they do it their own way, ignoring the hegemony of Tinder (50 million users), Grindr, Hinge and Minge. Or the temptation to 'Netflix and chill' just because everyone else will.

But some singletons I know have capitulated, and go on the hunt in the established manner, though many of them would agree with Zac Efron (the sage) that 'dating is kind of hard. Like dinner or something. Like a forced awkward situation.[60]' What could be more awkward than dinner?

This second set of single friends tell me how fraught it all is. They say they never know what they'll get on date night: creeps they've had to kick into touch with reality; men who've become mates but not in the animal kingdom sort of way; and the very occasional Adonis, whose seeming perfection they cannot vouch for with any certainty because they're rarely there for scrutiny in the morning. They recount all the effort that goes into the weekly conflux with relish: casting their nets far and wide to make a catch, chatting non-stop with friends for advice in the run-up to date night, the scramble to find the right push-up bra and tummy tucking underpants, the quick hoover round the flat in case there's a post-date *nightcap*, and the last minute handbag inventory for mace and should the fella turn out non-creepy, other equally important forms of protection. Frenzied, huh?

Hey, it's equally frenetic for us settled sorts. Don't be fooled by Smug Marrieds and the picture of cool, composed contentment they project. Pencilling in 'couple time' amidst the chaos, cacophony and the clamour for cuddles makes it every bit as complicated a mating ritual as that of single folk. There is that holding-your-breath excitement too, but not because you don't know what Cupid will bring. It's what the stork has already brought you that matters, and whether said Gifts From Stork plan to let you out!

Where single ladies might slave for hours, even weeks, to get the desired look, the mien the married mom of two will aim for is, well, just clean. With the husband home and the kids diverted temporarily, I throw on whatever I can find (which Hubby obligingly assures me looks brill). Before we can step out though, the bath will spring a leak and the pot roast explode in the kitchen. However, a minute's mop-up later (we've got good at this, much better than we are at making out), with the children entrusted to a reliable sitter, we are finally able to hit the road.

Where singleton sex (as differentiated from solo sex, a whole different hand game) really diverges from married mating is in the after-date action. I'm afraid you'll always have to take your husband home (unless he's been hugely obnoxious, in which case shouldn't you be considering divorce?). But you'll never have to reach for the mace or kitchen knife or worry about catching anything other than a cold (if you do, as above, right?). You will both reach for the key. You won't tear each other's clothes off in the hallway because the babysitter's waiting. Then it's cherubs before carnality, as you look in on your sleeping children before moving on to the things that produced them in the first place. But will you both be able to stay awake long enough to hit those high notes?

There is a touch more coitus as the children grow. You're less likely to find spaghetti splodges in your bed (unless you like being slathered in it; I prefer chocolate sauce myself). Your bits aren't aching unless it's to get fondled. Your body has also got back to its original shape and size, increasing your agility as well as your enthusiasm immensely. But now your children are always around the corner asking questions. And as every parent knows, kids' queries must be answered immediately or they multiply in volume, complexity and insistence like Gremlins fed at midnight. So, hiding hard-ons and hickies, you address pressingly urgent issues like the size of Santa's sleigh, how long is a piece of string and the girth of a unicorn's horn (even as your own shrinks in dismay). Not things that will occur to the single person set on a torrid tumble. Questions when caught up in the whirligig of lust are generally along the lines of, 'You got the condoms (prosaic but essential)?' or 'Do you love me (romantic, but potentially show-stopping)?'

If they're older, it's not that different a routine, only it's not the babysitter you have to clear off the premises but suitors of their own. And instead of angelic sleeping faces you might have smirky/sulky/sarky ones to deal with before you've finally shut that bedroom door. But then the rewards multiply if you've managed to get that far. I don't mean just that particular night; I mean, if you've got through that many years together and can still end up panting for each other after a great night out, then not only do you deserve congratulations but every sensual delight that awaits you in your boudoir.

So, does this battle of the sexes (married vs single) have a winner?

1. **Frequency**. Sex after marriage, especially after children, is *not* like life after death – it does happen! But it requires effort. Yet, don't we also know that safe, happy singleton sex isn't that easy to come by either, especially for the vast majority of normal folk, sometimes shy, rarely super-model material, living non-jet-setting lives? Despite all the freedoms and the apps, the American Sexual Behaviour Study found that single people have less sex than married couples! Partly because it's on tap for us married folks whether we get the chance to lap it up or not (not, generally, if you throw children into the mix). Other surveys suggest that millennials, usually unmarried, are making plenty of whoopee, but these are frequently based on age rather than marital status. And age is very definitely a factor in terms of, no, not how much you're getting but how much you *want*.
2. **Intensity**. Sex for the marrieds is rarely frantic (unless we're worried the kids will barge in, which happens A LOT). Also, neither of us is going anywhere, so there's no need for frenzy. But that actually makes it rather beautiful, in a languid, assured, slowly sensual way. And because we know the other well, we can't seriously goof up. Unless, in a moment of mid-life madness, we try to introduce something entirely novel like a new orifice to explore. Or GoT role-play (When she said she wanted stark? She meant naked).
3. **Creativity.** Couples who have made that commitment to hang together can let it all hang out without worry. No need after all for artfully arranged pillows to hide the podge they've already seen. So much easier then to try a new position or a sex toy that makes you wobble in places that shouldn't. But who cares? He's already

seen, touched and tasted your every swell. Yes, says the singleton, but with us *every body* is new and we don't need tricks and props to make it hot. You've got a point there, mate.

4. **Familiarity.** What singletons have with their myriad new partners is mystery, surprises (not always good), and a skin-prickling, even pant-wetting kind of frisson. But let's be honest, it's the anticipation that's exciting; reality is much less so. That's when the bespoke skill that comes with knowing your body well really matters. Your long-term partner will know from experience (all those hundreds of times you've reminded him) exactly which breast to fondle, which shoulder enjoys the occasional nip, whether you like your toes being sucked at all or a lazy tongue trailed up your thigh before that all-important plunge into Narnia. This is the *inside track* that comes with time spent doing each other. And you're on your way to as monumental an orgasm as any night with a newbie can give you.

Orgasm Smorgasm

Yet, despite the smorgasbord of partners and pleasures available, when it comes to orgasms, there aren't enough out there. Oh, men have plenty but they can get to 'third base' with just 'warm apple pie' (according to *American Pie*. And could a film that deep be wrong?). 75 per cent of men always reach orgasm during sex (making me awfully sorry for the unfortunate 25 per cent denied that pleasure). But only 29 per cent of women are so lucky. Most women don't climax through vaginal intercourse at all, needing clitoral stimulation instead. Single women with access to more partners (more chances to get it right, you'd think) experienced only marginally more orgasms than their hitched sisters (55 per cent orgasmed on half the occasions they had sex, compared to 48 per cent). 43 per cent of *all* women, single or married, have reported having trouble with reaching a climax[61].

And it's all down to giving her at least some of what she wants. But what does the sisterhood want in the sack? You scratch your head in mock terror and bafflement. So, I thought I'd be nice and do it for you instead – the asking. I said to my girlfriends, 'Tell me what you want, what you really, really want.'

Girlfriends: 'I wanna, I wanna, I wanna, I wanna really, really, really wanna zigazig ah.'

And it all made sense (more than the Spice Girls ever did). But let me spell it out for you. When it comes to the Big Girlie O, it isn't about Sporty, Spicy, Scary, Ginger or Posh. Oh, maybe just a little, in terms of approaches men could take. The women you really need to keep in mind are the three kinds on this planet when it comes to orgasms: satisfied, indulgent and frustrated.

1. **Satisfied Women.** They have genuine orgasms and not just that once in 1949. That year, apparently, sexually satisfied women were particularly thin on the ground with one woman capturing the sexual zeitgeist with, 'If only he would make love to me instead of using me like a chamber pot.[62]' Unfortunately, that was not the last bad year for female orgasms as current statistics demonstrate. Women continue to be made to feel like repositories for emissions, getting piss-poor pleasure out of it themselves. But there *are* sensitive men out there and women who've found them. They are the lucky 29 per cent; our Satisfied (or considering how rare it is, Super-Satisfied) Sistuhs.

2. **Indulgent Women.** These know their men are trying very hard, but sadly without the desired effect, and not wanting to see grown men cry, have become au fait at fauxgasms. Like Meg Ryan in *When Harry Met Sally*, they groan with abandon and throw themselves about as if they'd just discovered a chocolate-slathered Tom Hiddleston between their legs. She deserved an Oscar and so do they, having pulled off this performance, not once but every friggin' night of their lives. And their men know they've got to pull their finger out (and in and ...) if they want payback. So, they keep trying, and their women live in hope.
3. **Frustrated Women**: 62 percent of women worldwide are said to be dissatisfied with their sex lives. In Japan, 45 per cent of them have sworn off sex altogether. And in India, divorces initiated by women are up 10 per cent because they won't put up with ineptitude (in bed and out) from their men anymore. These women are neither satisfied nor indulgent because their men won't even *try* to please them in bed. Instead they surf tirelessly for porn (42 per cent of American men and up to 93 per cent of young Indian men allegedly find porn addictive), drool over Bollywood babes/ladsmag models and leer at women in passing. But when it comes to the woman at home, they can't muster up the interest to actually, properly, make love to her. What's the deal, gentlemen? Exhausted from hours of intensive wanking? Afraid of real intercourse with a real woman?

As a real woman who's had real intercourse with some proper orgasms along the way, maybe I can help. Perhaps I could provide some pointers on what women want?

1. **Skill.** And sensitivity. When it comes to making love to a woman, they go hand in hand (hands being the operative word, capisce?). As Bryan Adams said, 'To really love a woman, let her hold you, till you know how she needs to be touched, you've gotta breathe her, really taste her,' etc. All good advice from a Man Who Knows. You see, for the female of the species, foreplay and not penetration is key to the climax. For her, it is very often the most important element of the whole experience. As the American sex educator Betty Dodson declared, 'Intercourse is okay. But I much prefer a talented tongue on my clitoris.[63]' And who doesn't love pie? Dig in, gentlemen.
2. **Stamina.** Women can be at it for much longer and in fact, need longer at it to get there. The average man, however, rarely lasts as long in the sack (anything from forty-four seconds to five minutes) but can train himself to make it to a deliciously long forty-four minutes (really, it's not just Sting). This makes the average woman rather happy. Not only because it's evidence of effort on their behalf, but sexually satisfied folk are known to be healthier, happier folk. And it's just mind over matter, guys. Yes, *that* matter, between your legs. So why does it seem not to matter to so many men?

   Obviously it is embedded in culture *everywhere* that not only are women disinterested in sex (or should be), their satisfaction, in just about everything, matters less than that of men. In some countries, this bs has hung around longer than others. And so foreplay is reputed to last twenty minutes longer in the West (irrespective of the ethnicity of those involved), with men more likely to go down on their women.

But there is biology as well. Men and women appear designed to almost never meet in the middle in a mutually satisfactory way. Women hit their sexual peak in their mid-thirties when they are supposed to be past their sell-by-date and have been put out to pasture in favour of apparently more desirable, much younger women (who haven't often matured enough physically to really enjoy sex). Men, on the other hand, reach their optimum sexual age at a juvenile seventeen. More than 40 per cent of men over the age of forty experience erectile dysfunction. And propping them up with Viagra is risky. If he dies in the saddle, *you'll* never ride again!

But if the only men capable of keeping up with us sexually are the gangling, acne-ridden teenage boys we'd rather dunk (in antiseptic) than bonk, and society actively opposes (with the endearing exception of Emmanuel Macron) these cougar-toy boy couplings designed to deliver the greatest sexual satisfaction anyway, then what is the answer?

3. Is it multiple lovers we need then? Men have their harems. On the sly. In their fevered imaginations. But they don't actually require them. They do need strings of women but only to service their shaky egos. Women, however, last longer, need more stimulation and can multitask, which can be too much for one man to handle. And didn't our very own epic mistress (boss, not concubine) of five warlike brothers show the way? The swashbuckling heroine of India's greatest epic was one sassy lady who successfully managed a male harem long before Indian women had been browbeaten into believing that an embarrassment of orgasmic riches was for men alone.

Or are sex toys the answer? 'I didn't enjoy sex till I started masturbating.' Eva Longoria revealed. 'I bought my first vibrator three years ago and now I give vibrators to all my girlfriends. They scream when they get it (and ever after) because the best gift I can give them is an orgasm.[64]' Still, sex toys without someone to play with? Limitless fun, but no cuddles after? And some of us, inexplicably, prefer men. The fumbling. The bumbling. The flesh-and-blood boner. Many of us even want just the one.

But it *is* about numbers in the end: the number of times you do each other, the number of years you spend making out together, and, as old-fashioned as it may sound, the affection you have for each other. That just makes you a little less selfish in bed, a little more attentive. And a lot more licky!

Twelve years after our wedding, there's still nothing like the morning after a married date night, despite the fatigue, the not-quite mint-condition bodies, and that wee bit of missing frisson you admittedly get with a new man. When the sun creeps up to your bed instead of the children (what has the babysitter fed them, you wonder), he's still there beside you, the man you love. He feels you stirring, smiles and says in that deep Yorkshire voice that still turns you on, 'You are the most beautiful thing I have ever seen.'

'Still?' you ask, to check he's wide awake and in possession of his senses.

'Still,' he says, as he draws you into his arms again, 'and that will never change.'

But even as I open my legs to revisit those delicious sensations we've discovered together over the years, I cross my fingers tightly under the sheets.

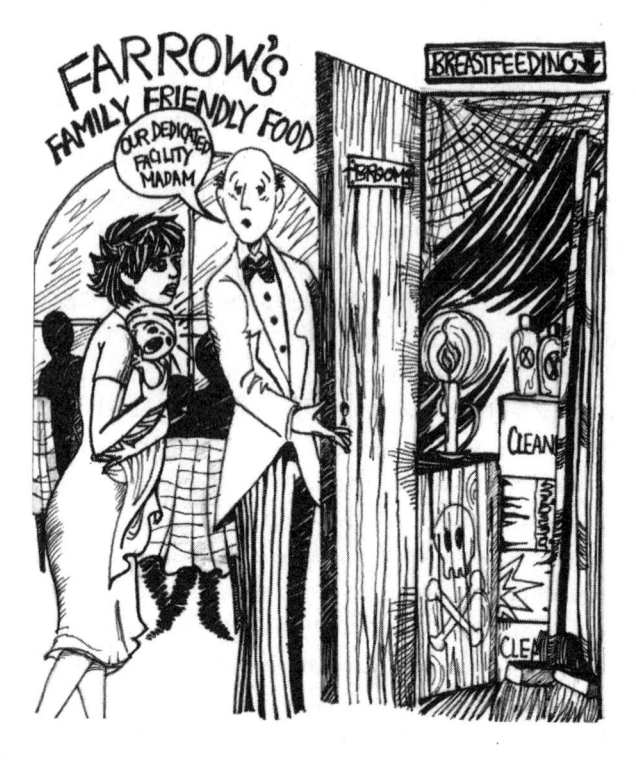

14

The Bouncy, Baleful World of Binky and Bonky

Ah, the history of a woman's breasts, how they sprout, grow, defy gravity for decades only to go swiftly south thereafter. But, before that, how they respond to touch, get heavy with milk when the consequences of that touch knock us up (so, I've skipped a few steps in between), and then sometimes, sadly, develop bumps of a nature that are not the stuff of perky songs ('my bumps, my bumps, my lovely lady lumps' suddenly sounds so wrong).

These can cause great distress, lead to invasive or debilitating treatment and sometimes, death. So, the story of a woman's breasts is often the story of the woman as a physical being. Like it or not (and there's a lot not to like), the path our bodies plot through this world is frequently directed, very often derailed and sometimes brought to a standstill by our Twin Balls of Uncertain Benefit.

The story of my boobs starts with having none for the longest time. I had neither breasts nor many girlfriends (a loner with my nose in books, when I did make friends with another misfit, it was usually a boy). When the two or three girls I was closest to started wearing training bras with great pride, and began to look like women at around twelve or thirteen, I still looked six and did not need any support at all. On top of which, unlike my friends, I really didn't like the idea of having to wear them (and still wriggle out of them now – literally – as often as I can). This could have been because of the misshapen horrors my mother would buy for herself from the fashion-crime haven of Gariahat Market. Or it might have been quite the reverse; that aesthetics didn't matter as I was a fiery, bra-burning feminist in the making already. But then they did appear, budding from midge-bites to molehills nearly three years after everyone else, and swelling to mountains (but British ones, not the Himalayas) decades later. With it came pressure to pin mine down with those pectoral pouches Bengali women called 'beh-raa'. Not to be confused with bhera, though we *are* sheep-like in our acceptance of these imposed physical restraints.

Indian bras back then were not meant to make you feel

feminine, sensuous or swish; they felt like punishment, and I do believe they were meant to be. Punishment for being a woman, for developing things as incendiary as breasts and then having the temerity to suggest we could decide what happened to them. That couldn't be allowed, of course. No, we must hide our WMD's, and punish our impertinence in growing them by tormenting our tainted flesh with ugly, chafing constraints. That was the point of bras in 1980s India.

There was no getting out of it, however. By the time I started at a new school at sixteen, a co-ed for my last two years of schooling, I was the proud possessor of several of those crumpled, conical horrors my mother favoured, shaped to fit no human breast ever, and without the effrontery of Madonna's exaggerated cones from the nineties. But the white shirts at this new school were thin and went sheer in the heavy monsoon rains. If you avoided getting caught in the rains, you were bound to be splashed by cars or rampaging children (and sometimes purposeful older boys) as you waded through thigh-high water in the narrow lanes outside the school. And so I began to wear bras, grudgingly.

All these years later and half a world away, my relationship with bras hasn't changed much, even though I now have many beautiful, luxurious, sensuous ones to choose from. I have two drawers full of them; lacy, peek-a-boo ones; sporty, practical ones; and bras with sassy candy pink trim or winking black sequins. I've got plush plum-coloured brassieres as well as plain cotton virgin-whites. I even have a fur trimmed one for Christmas and a coconut shell pair for laughs. They are silky, satiny, velvety and all so comfortable that they could be second skin.

A few of my bras show acres of cleavage; others a flash of caramelicious side-boob while some modestly reveal just a hint of swell. I now have lingerie for every reason, season and mood. I have bras that make me feel mumsy, others decidedly sexy and some that are gird-up-my-globes-and-get-on-with-the-day-eey. But this treasure trove of jewel-bright jug ornaments took a long time coming, and by then I'd made up my mind I didn't care to wear them.

For a girl whose periods started at eleven, I had to wait an eternity to be recognized as a woman because breasts (to men certainly) are what set women apart from girls. Breasts, boobs, jugs, melons, baps, titties, knockers – those globes of apparently wildly desirable fat, make the world go round, it's clear (and sad). I should know! For years there wasn't a bump in sight, but once they grew, a whole section of the population started behaving differently towards me. Older men got censorious. Younger ones polarized into the bashful or predatory. Men of all ages suddenly had the licence to cop a feel on the sly. Brushing against my boobies as if unaware, even reaching out and squeezing them if sufficiently concealed by a big, jostling crowd (the Pujos they deemed best for this activity, between piously offering prayers to the Devi and going home to self-righteously demand lunch from their wives). All this because breasts – real ones, as opposed to celluloid – aren't generally available to men in India. None for single men and only the lone pair for the married, which they tire of quickly. With breasts becoming more available, at least more visually accessible, with the opening up of India in the nineties, you might have hoped that Indian men would turn over a new, blasé and therefore, restrained leaf. But no. The unasked-for fondling continues unabated.

This unsolicited fumbling on buses eased somewhat when I could afford to get taxis, which didn't stop the getting-felt-up in large crowds and tight spaces though. And the solicited fondling on trains started. Oh, okay, it happened just the once. And once on the television studio floor. On the sofa of my little house in Sheffield. And that time under the ... you know it all now really. My breasts did see a little more action than Vee did because of my predilection for going so far and no further (knowing when to stop I called it, cocktease, fumed the boys).

As I grew older and more poised and was subjected to fewer fumbles, my breasts perked up and developed a personality. No, sorry, *individual* personalities. One breast was more outgoing (always ready to pop out), keen to be touched (it strained towards men I liked, no kidding); it was the first to fill up with milk and first to get sore she wasn't being suckled exclusively. A bit of a diva. The other was more thoughtful and, as a result, more prone to gloom (occasionally given to drooping), more of a shrinking violet (but not violet, no, not a vein to be seen after two years of breastfeeding if I do say so myself), less keen on the sucking (from man or baby) and consequently, less likely to give me grief over the musical breasts situation (oh, you know the game you play with Baby where they stubbornly resist one in favour of the other, more beloved boob, even as you try everything to move them on). This was the understudy.

So, my breasts were crying out for names. I already had Wanda and Vee. So, the shyer one I called Binky, rhyming with slinky (off into the shadows), blinky with surprise at finding herself in the spotlight, etc. The bouncier one was, therefore, Bonky. She so clearly enjoyed romps more.

Bonky (loud stage whisper): Go on, get in there.

Binky (whispering): No, um, you go.

Bonky: Oh, don't be a wuss, you'll enjoy it.

Binky (hanging her head, as she did): They can be rough and ...

But before she could finish telling her twin about her reservations, an exasperated (and excited) Bonky had launched herself into the firm grasp of Waiting Man, without so much as a by-your-leave from me. Bonky led from the front in all things, scything through crowds like Moses parting the Red Sea (how pleased the pious will be with that comparison). Binky, encouraged by her perkier partner, would usually fall in step and I would sail through motley masses from Times Square to Tollygunge with some ogling, but no resistance at all. Growing them wasn't all bad after all. They opened so many doors, sometimes literally, I had grown quite attached to them (not that I had a choice).

But when I told my friends I'd named them just like my children (I may have omitted to tell them I'd named my womb and woof too), they asked if I had a favourite breast. Of course not, I protested. Like my kids, they were both sources of pleasure and vexation in equal measure. And pain. Both had been loved, squeezed, twisted and deliberately hurt. They had also driven me to distraction with their dripping, peeping and flipping. But if I didn't have a favourite, others with a claim on them certainly did.

Baby #1 practically came out of the womb roaring for his favourite breast, which was not unsurprisingly, Bonky. Of course, I'd been told not to allow single-breast-fixated feeding. Of course, I tried to dissuade him, even slathering Bonky's chocolate brown nipple with bright banana-yellow baby food (which Baby had turned his nose up at earlier). But on his favourite breast he loved it! In the end, he settled down to suckling both but always with a soft spot for bouncy

Bonky. I already knew that Daddy had a preference for Bonky, wrapping his tongue around her as often over the years as Baby #1 in his first year.

Only Baby #2, my little girl, showed a preference for bashful Binky (ah, the girl child, always sees what others can't) and Binky blossomed in the warmth of her attention. She would seek out Binky, snuggle up to her, falling asleep every night pillowed on Binky's sudden vastness. As for the dude on the street, he was a democratic fella, as long as he got a gander at one or BOTH, he was happy.

But have breasts worked for *you*?

1. They are attention-getters. That's good when you get the last seat on the train and a hand with the luggage. But not-so-good when the minute you take that seat and accept a hand, they think you want to be handled too.
2. They are unmanageable, like hair, slipping out of whatever they've been squished into, peeping out at inopportune moments. They even go hard, pointy and very noticeable under our clothes (though never as much as the easy-up tent poles that men have) when cold, frightened, aroused or angry. On the bright side, while men everywhere become transfixed by nothing more than two little bobbles of flesh showing through clothing, you could rob Fort Knox and they wouldn't know it.
3. They get in the way of activities, from running to cooking. Boobs, especially big ones, are a hindrance rather than a help. Unless you consider a swift dip of breast that's not chicken breast into your cooking an enhancement. Luckily, there are at least two activities for which they are an advantage.

4. Sex being the first one. Most men like big ones so it follows that having mammoths (no, I don't, I'm just generalizing. And no I won't let you be the judge) means more nookie. If you're footloose, fancy-free and looking for a different partner every night, the size of your melons may well drive up activity. But for women in relationships, sleeping with the same man nightly, it is the size of our yawn rather than the circumference of our jugs that will determine the likelihood of sex that night.
5. While on the subject of the part our breasts play in what passes as foreplay, let's once and for all make what NOT to do to them man-clear. Please let's not have any more pinching, biting, or that, ugh, icky-sicky-leave-drool-on-the-nippy slurping. And for f*** sake, stop squeezing them like balls of dough! We love a man who bakes but our baps ain't for kneading. Expert licking and sucking though – do carry on!
6. Sucking and suckling are worlds apart, but confuse the pervy and the prudish (who are often the same). I've found to my horror that that's why some women fight shy of feeding their own babies. But it isn't remotely alike! The feelings that well up in me (along with the milk) when Baby is at my breast are nothing like the flip-flops in my tummy when a man's at work. It's like stopping eating because it reminds you of fellatio. Just. Plain. Weird. Breastfeeding, for me, has undoubtedly been one of the benefits of having breasts. Holding that velvety, fuzzy thing you've brought into the world as close as can be and feeding it from your own body is a strangely wonderful and overwhelmingly emotional experience. And that's besides all the good it does.

Breastfed children are six times more likely to survive the early months than bottle-fed kids. It supports the child's brain development too, and is associated with bigger academic strides at the primary level. It also protects children from disease in later years. It does the mother good as well, lessening the likelihood of post-partum haemorrhage right away and type 2 diabetes, breast, uterine and ovarian cancer in the future[65]. It made me feel like the centre of the universe; giver of life and nourishment. But there are snags.

The Three Bees

Bonking leads to **B**abies (often) and babies lead to **B**reastfeeding (less often; only 23 per cent of British and 27 per cent of US moms breastfeed for any length of time, although heart-warmingly, and probably out of necessity, 92 per cent of Indian mothers breastfeed their babies for the first twelve months).

With Baby's arrival, both bonking and Vee hung up their boots. Wanda retired hurt too. Even Baby, after lapping up the adulation and all the milk it could get its tiny balled fists on, just got on with growing. The spotlight then shifted almost completely to my heavy milk-laden breasts. Nobody, other than family and medical staff, could be bothered with Wanda or even Vee once pregnant, but everyone and their uncle seemed keen on my outrageously swollen breasts. And those perennially wet nipple patches. No day was complete without a peek down my décolletage (man) or a surmise on how Baby was feeding (woman).

But all the time your brimming-over breasts are being viewed by men as a manifestation of overflowing sexuality, you know that in fact it's the opposite. While Baby's feeding, there'll be no breeding (plenty of bad rhyming though). Not least because Vee was still raw from everything she'd been through or more accurately, everything that had been through her. Wanda, in the meantime, had gone into a deep sleep and with her, my sex drive. Love I felt biologically obliged to withhold too from all but my babies in those early stages. And with Baby (each in their turn) drinking prodigiously and (what felt like) continuously, both sleep and lovemaking went out the window. Disappearing with a dejected sigh into the heart of Sherwood.

Of the two, if I'm honest, sleep was the more desirable. Sleep is the holy grail, the pot 'o gold at the end of the rainbow, the treasure chest buried beneath the sea for the breastfeeding mom – a longed-for impossibility. Because if Baby isn't keeping her up, her aching, leaking hormonal breasts are.

Bonky: I need a long, lingering cocoa butter massage.

Binky: Shhhh. Let her sleep. She hasn't in weeks.

Bonky: A warm, foamy bubble-bath? She can have a bubble bath asleep, can't she?

Binky (ever the practical one): But who'll run it? You like being handled but are you handy?

Mutter, mutter, mutter went Bonky, which equated to a sore and jumpy breast that wouldn't let me sleep yet again. Breasts can indeed be hormonal and temperamental, especially before or after birth or when you're breastfeeding. They change temperature, have nervy tics jumping in them, heated blood surges to and fro. They can also grow hard, bumpy, ridiculously painful and seem about to burst like overripe fruit. And it can all happen in the blink of an eye or over excruciating days of discomfort. It's called puerperal mastitis and affects one in ten breastfeeding women. I had it bad.

To start with, neither Baby nor I knew how to breastfeed. Baby would take my nipple in its mouth and then let go, unable to hold on. I would keep sticking that boob back in like I'd been instructed, not changing breast till I'd exhausted the possibilities of the first. Baby would turn away stubbornly or cry to signify unwillingness (no one had ever done that before!). When even the other breast was rejected, it would be my turn to cry. If it was the right time of day, I would collect myself and call the mid-wife to bombard her with questions. Baby was having trouble latching on, I would yelp. Most babies did, she would counter. I was a resolute mom, she went on to reassure, and must keep on trying.

But all the good advice in the world didn't help till almost the end of that first week when Bonky, the diva, the troublesome one, suddenly made it all fall into place. As I lay down, trying a new position with Baby to help it feed (and because my back hurt from all the unlikely suckling stances I'd tried, including arching back while standing up), Bonky bounced into Baby's maw at a completely new angle. Sweet, warm milk squirted into its mouth, sliding down its throat comfortingly instead of hitting the back as it usually did with the force of a fireman's hose. Baby gurgled happily and latched on firmly for the first time. And we were away.

As Baby blossomed, I felt vindicated in having stuck to my guns. But as soon as my confusion over Baby's apparent reluctance to feed had cleared, along came other hurdles, mostly socially constructed ones.

My decision to breastfeed meant that Binky, Bonky and Baby were the centre of my existence for a short, but draining period. Wherever I went, these hefty appendages came with me. And Baby I couldn't leave at home either.

Not only did I not have family living nearby to leave my babies with, I didn't really want to, because I genuinely enjoyed their company. But that meant having to feed them out and about. I soon found myself plopping my puppies (and I don't mean the children) on to restaurant tables, park-bench armrests and car trays, all as hygienically as possible, and even slightly shielded. What I hadn't factored in was the hysteria surrounding breastfeeding outside of the smallest cupboard in the darkest room of your house, where society wants to put nursing women.

From aged relatives to medical professionals to powder milk lobbyists, everyone will tell you what to do with your lactating breasts, when and how. You *should* feed your baby breast milk, we are told, because it contains antibodies and nutrients essential for their health and development, which cannot be reproduced artificially. And most of us would agree. But you must also never let anyone see you do it. EVER. Like Medusa's gaze, a glimpse of nipple will turn men to stone (and not just down there apparently) and some women stony with disapproval. So, breastfeeding moms, beware; you're a public safety hazard and must not be let out of doors. Just before you hide away in the dark forever though, let them have a long, lingering look down your deep, delish plunging mommy cleavage, no?

No.

My baby daughter made the arduous annual journey to India before she was three months old. My little boy made what felt like an equally endless journey to Chateaubriand in France by car when he was three months old too. On the flight to India, with Indian passengers of a certain vintage (with years of tsk-tsking behind them), I accepted I'd have to conceal myself while feeding, behind the endlessly snaking scarf I'd brought with me. And because Baby fed so often, I soon gave up dismantling my makeshift tent, spending the rest of the flight in its dark depths.

'Won't you come out?' entreated my husband.

'I cannot see the scratchers, snorers and dribblers. I am staying put.'

'Can I come in?' he said.

I had expected to have to conceal my breastfeeding on an Indian flight. What really shocked me was the 'liberal' western world's approach to it. In France, which is all 'ooh la la' and 'c'est la vie' and anything goes, I had to leave the café I was dining in with my family to hide away in our car like a Calais-bound immigrant to feed my baby. As Baby fed often, my most enduring memory of charming Normandy was being cooped up in the sedan with him suckling hungrily (but also losing great gulps of it down the front of my new chic Parisian top). As the car's interiors smelt of nappies and milk, I had rolled down the window to the cool night air and can still remember a song wafting from somewhere, alluringly conjuring up images of tangles in the backs of old Renaults that did not involve, unlike mine, a baby.

But then the street lamps flickered and, when I heard a thunderclap, I scooted back in to where the family was dining. Thunderstorms didn't scare me, but wasting my life being a decorous mother did. I finished my steak that night, and my crème brulee, while Baby was kept entertained by the rest of the family. After that incident, I refused to do the patriarchal thing of hiding away like a felon while performing the most natural function in the world. Till I was compelled to, and in the most unlikely place.

On our return from France that year, I started to unfurl my feeding wings, first nursing in relatively secluded public spots partially covered by a coat, to openly wherever necessary, buses, tram stops, not-especially-sheltered park benches and busy sidewalk cafes. I wore my suckling baby like a badge of courage to encourage other moms to do the same. Till I tried it in an English hospital that trumpeted how much it cared: 'Here for mothers and babies!' In this hospital, where they bombarded you constantly with the benefits of breastfeeding, I was told to cover up and move along when, in a quiet corner of their paediatric waiting room, I tried to feed my baby.

'What do you think you're doing?'

'Er, feeding my baby.'

'You can't do that! What do you think this is – a hippie commune? A naturist beach? Your loo?'

'No,' I said, 'I think it is the paediatric waiting room of a hospital that screams the benefits of breastfeeding at every turn and should set an example when it comes to allowing feeding mothers to go about their business unhindered.'

But that dragon of a nurse, who was muttering disgustedly to herself, was too busy frogmarching us like naughty children to a dark, musty room with barely a stick of furniture, to hear me. There, amidst the timorous light and mouldy fumes, balanced on a rickety table, I was meant to feed my baby, hidden away from the other patients who would apparently be shocked and upset at such a sight.

Stunned at this treatment coming from the British National Health Service, which campaigns to bring breastfeeding back to the UK in a big way, I gave them another earful and left. I should have done more. But breastfeeding had ironically left me too drained to take up the cudgels for breastfeeding. Still, if it's worth anything to you, here's the ditty I used to sing when censorious glares and ogling stares impinged on me as I breastfed out and about. To the tune of Billy Joel's *'My life'*, ladies, here it is:

'I don't need you to tell me how to bring Baby up right,
I won't have you tell me I must feed her at home,
I don't care what you say anymore, this is my life,
Get your mitts off my breasts and leave my baby alone.'

Belt it out and watch dirty old men and meddlesome biddies scatter, if for no other reason than they think you're mad. You also get that extra bit of elbow room and breathing space you need to feed Baby for a brief but happy while. And maybe, just maybe, somebody actually gets the message too. I stuck it out, both with the breastfeeding and the occasional singing-to-shoo-the-sods-away. Looking at my kids now, it feels well worth the pains and pariah-hood.

Then one day, Baby was ready to move on to solids and Binky and Bonky were demoted from Very Important Parts of the body to peripheral players. It was not just a metaphorical loss of stature either. They shrank to half the size they had been. Baby was distraught. They had been weaned off mommy milk little by little, but now they weren't being given their favourite breast at all, replaced by the cold comforts of bottle or beaker and clothed cuddles. If Baby was unhappy, so was Mommy, but for other reasons too. I had got used to my new body, its large, luscious Earth Mother contours. It was a new kind of sexy I hadn't known before, and the ogling was a small annoyance compared to the mother goddess potency I felt, which went beyond mere looks.

But then, I relished the prospect of having my old svelte self back, and getting on with a new stage of life for Baby. One in which we were both more independent and less breast-absorbed. More sleep and less pain too, I imagined happily. However, this was not to be. I did not get my old body back, nor my sleep. What I saw in the mirror after gave me a shock.

Underneath my vastly diminished breasts was a sad, little sack like a colostomy bag. When did I sign up for this, I thought? But I hadn't. That was my stomach. It had lost all shape in the course of two pregnancies and two deliveries, one of which involved over a day of labour. After all that stretching, pulling and pushing, my tummy had as much chance of turning the clock back to taut, as the earth had to pre-industrial purity.

To add insult to injury, it was also riven by railway track scars criss-crossing it in a desperate hurry to get somewhere. Anywhere. Anywhere off that horror of a tummy. I almost couldn't bear looking further, but as I walked away from the mirror (with elaborate plans of gagging, cuffing and hauling it into the loft for its sins), I couldn't help but catch sight of bigger thighs and a spreading bottom too.

So, you try to whip yourself back into shape (whip is right as it involves such a lot of self-flagellating discipline and hawk-eyed hate of oneself). But without a round-the-clock regime (or the time for one) and an entourage comprising personal trainer, shopper, dietician, masseuse and clown (to cheer you up when the rigours get you down), most ordinary women don't stand a chance of getting their pre-baby bodies back. Then you run a bit longer and eat ice cream fewer times in the day (i.e., not every time you're blue), and you get back an approximation of what you had.

The stomach looks like a stomach again and not a colostomy bag (though never again like a washboard either). The thighs and bottom have shrunk, making the breast-bottom ratio proportionate once more. Binky had even perked up a bit (jogged into pertness from all that exercise). How does it matter, you might ask? Yet, you know it does. Not because you care what the man on the street, the catty woman next door or the fashion mags say.

But brought up in this world as you have been (and not on some progressive planet where you're all soul and little bulk), you care about what you see in the mirror and how it makes you feel. You care about slipping into attractive clothes rather than squeezing into them. You care about going for a swim unselfconsciously. Most of all, you care about not being out of puff constantly. And being around a long, long time for those you love. You've worked at it, you've got back some of your mojo, and you couldn't be more pleased. But then you notice with a sinking feeling that other things have begun to give. There are waggling bags of flesh under your arms and your knees look knobblier than Santa's sack.

Then you know it's time. Time to do what you always meant to. Go topless on the beach. Go topless in the park in summer. Haggle bare-chested in the market on muggy afternoons. Sit gossiping with the girls, all nipples-free, as the asphalt melts on the streets. Men do it all the time. Men do it because it's hot, because it's not and because they think their wobbling moobs and bulging gut turn women on. Of course men can strip and it isn't nudity. It isn't indecent, immoral or illegal. But a woman stripping to cool off can send the world into a tizzy. It could only be allowed in lewd and carnal corners of the world – nudist beaches, naturist communes or the dark feral dens of feeding moms.

Now that you have nothing to lose (having lost elasticity, conventional allure, inhibitions and face), it's time to hoist your flag (and your top) for womankind and the never-ending fight for equal rights. Because you aren't pert and ripe for the picking any more (not to the conventionally blinkered; precisely the kind you don't want to appeal to), you can let it all hang out without a worry about playing into their hands (in every sense). Plus, that fearsome scowl you wear as you worry distractedly about career, children and the plugged drains at home will protect you better than clothes ever did.

In Canada, female toplessness was legalized in the new millennium. In the US, baring breasts for breastfeeding 'on federal property' was made legal in 1999. Many Western European nations are tolerant of topless women in selected settings[66]. But it remains sexualized, illegal or at least frowned upon in much of the world. In the Middle East, East Asia and even America, social proscriptions against bare breasts have actually been expanded to include prepubescent and infant girls recently.

Women, in turn, have been battling double standards bare-bodied for decades. In the sixties, women burnt bras in public places. More recently, semi-naked women have taken to the streets and the social media to protest inequities, from the Naked Rumps for Trump movement in the US in 2016 campaigning against his misogyny[67] to the Free the Nipple crusade on England's Brighton Beach in the same year where 200 women dropped their tops to de-sexualize breasts and normalize their nakedness in everyday settings[68]. Or the powerful protest by a dozen middle-aged women in Manipur in 2004, where they disrobed completely in front of an army stronghold to demonstrate against the rape and murder of a young local woman[69].

Such bare-bodied or topless protests against rape and sexual harassment have spread to Brazil, Belgium, South Africa and many more places in the world. Amongst more oppressed women, baring breasts may be a step too far, but they have been whipping off their hijabs and posting selfies online to make the same point; that our bodies are ours, as are *all* the decisions to do with them.

So, what say all us slightly worse-for-wear women hit the

streets, brazen, bare-breasted and badass? Besides striking a blow for women's equality, imagine how good you'll feel about your body all over again and it'll have nothing to do with whether the world deems you desirable or not. Because amidst all the protests, campaigns and revolutions you *should* partake of, there is one that should happen in the quiet of your own home (and when I say you, I mean me too). We need to learn to love our bodies more than men do. Before the world can accept without derision women's bodies changing through childbirth, disease and age, we need to embrace our own. If you love what you have, it's a matter of time before everyone else will.

To get the ball rolling, let me say this:

I love you, Vee and Wanda. Love you, Binky and Bonky. You go, girls.

15

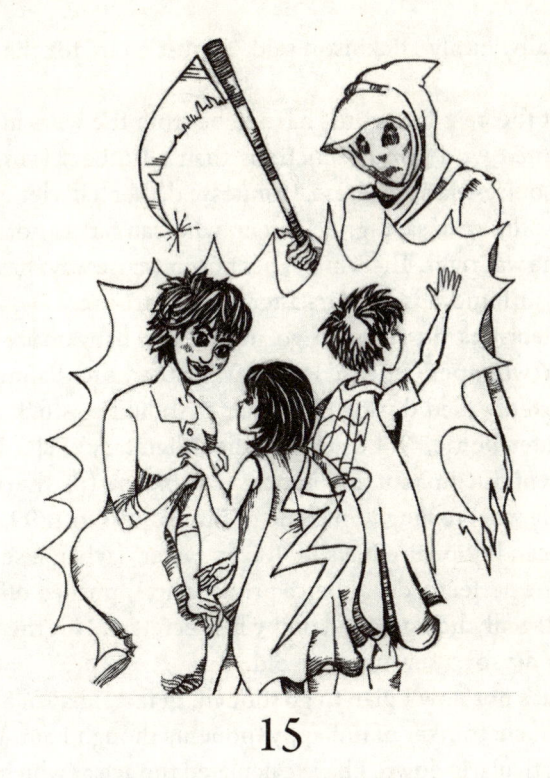

Death Rattles and Rolls On

Death rattles. It rattles me of late.

A death rattle is also the last sound a dying person makes, a gurgling, clicking, expiring sound, a giving up the ghost sound. But if you're lucky, you end life with a lot more than a rattle. Famous people have usually amassed far more, and have a thing or two to say too, before Curtain Call. Humphrey Bogart is believed to have told Lauren Bacall in his gruffly loving way, 'Goodbye Kid, hurry back.' More poetically, Emily Dickinson said, 'I must go in, for the fog is rising'.

But the best last words have to be from the woman more concerned with bodily functions than all others (yes, even me). Louise-Marie-Thérèse, Comtesse de Vercellis let one off right at the end, saying, 'A woman who can fart is not dead.' And she was right. The whiff of her no-nonsense ways has hung in the air hundreds of years after her de-fart-ure.

Celebrities do seem to go out with a bang more often than a whimper. British Prime Minister Lord Palmerston purportedly died during intercourse (should've stuck to the hot water bottle, M'Lord). Another 'dignitary' Felix Faure, President Incumbent of France, was blown (in the nicest possible way) to kingdom come by his mistress in 1899, while American billionaire Nelson 'Rocky Feller' (when else has a surname perfectly described a private part?) pushed off as he was allegedly being pulled off by his secretary. Not the worst way to die for a seventy-year-old.

That's not how I plan to go though. In fact, I haven't dwelt on it much, thinker of unhappy thoughts though I am. When I'm particularly down, I have calculated the age at which I can walk away from everything without affecting my kids. But I've always given us a good long run together with a gentle fading away after. Perhaps in my dotage, with both my family and faculties still about me, looking out at green hills rolling down to sparkling sea, my hands folded over the last engrossing book I shall ever read with a spur-of-the-moment mojito by my side. And cake. No death wish could be complete without cake. Or drowning in a vat of dark chocolate (yes, there's a sugary pattern here and it's diabetes I'll die of really).

Like the Duke of Clarence who was drowned at his request in a barrel of his favourite Malmsey Wine, having been sentenced to death for treachery by Edward IV. The best way to die he'd thought, but it turned out otherwise. Because drowning is not a dreamy floating away but a nasty, gargling, puking, lung-shattering, intensely painful death. By all accounts (clearly not from those who've succeeded). I think I'll pass. And sure, I like the idea of dying tangled in my lover's arms, but not in the act, frozen for posterity in some undignified posture (so, I like some of the more unusual ones, but it doesn't mean I want to be found that way). Ugh.

The truth is there's no such thing as a pleasant death. It is always unpleasant for someone. Unless you've pissed off everyone you ever knew (haven't done that *yet*, but who knows what this book might do). In the last few years, death has become more than disagreeable; it has been intimate in an unwelcome way. Alongside the losses of several friends and family members, was that of the baby I never knew. The repercussions rippled through my life for the next few years. Yet, the distressing fallout had less to do with death than learning, with great difficulty, how to negotiate *life*. All over again. As if life really did begin at forty!

This second wind now had an urgency about it. The pinpricks of mortality morphed into a steady rhythmic hammering that reminded me how much I had left to do. But what to do with what-to-do? Make a bucket list? Draft a will? Or pack everything you can into every precious day?

A will is for the morbidly afraid or the eminently sensible, neither of which I am. 47 per cent of British adults have a will with 30 per cent having drafted these before they turned thirty-five. 50 per cent of Americans with children have them too. And hey, I just remembered, so do I. Somewhere, and I have a good reason why. I made one when living in fear for my life during my divorce, because my ex-husband told me he would kill me rather than part with the house – half the house. He shoved me down the stairs to prove he meant it. I lived. And I bought the house. The WHOLE house. And I made a will because we were still married in the eyes of the law, which meant that another, more purposeful shove down the stairs would have given him everything I had worked so hard to secure. That will no longer applies (in case you're getting any ideas) and now in a gentler, happier world of my own making, I don't draft wills anymore. Or bucket lists. I am much too busy living. So why am I dwelling on death all of a sudden? Because my children are.

It all started with Rudolph on our yearly Yuletide trip to shabby, shambling, stunning Calke Abbey in the Derbyshire Dales. Not surprising, as so much of my life seemed to happen on those dales: that first marriage proposal, my first … er … non-solo orgasm, and now my children's annual encounter with Santa.

And this time, death …

Crunching up the lengthy, frosty drive, we found ourselves at the back of a long and winding line to see Santa. So we took ourselves off for our usual wander round the wintry park. At the kids' insistence (every year, I tell you) we covered further frigid ground to see the reindeers grazing in their large pen. They were, as always, miles away, and they always looked the same, but the kids loved them.

Buffeted by bone-chilling winds and knee-deep in mud, we enthusiastically pointed out Rudolph (but of course you can see him, we would chime *every* year – his nose glows as everyone knows!), and discussed the very important preparation for their long, long flight around the world on Christmas Eve.

Then, when we ran out of embellishments for the same

Christmas story we trotted out every year, and our teeth were chattering something awful, we steered them in for a spot of cocoa and meat pie. The food hall, a beamed barn, was heaving with goodies. That year we lighted on ranch-reared reindeer flan at a farm stall famous for their game pies. We took ours to a warm seat by the fireplace to apportion it amongst the four of us. Sinking our teeth into the steaming, spiced meat and fluffy pastry, we grown-ups looked around in satisfaction, only to notice that the two small faces opposite us were scrunched up in concern.

'Is that Rudolph in this pie, Mommy?' Our daughter asked.

'No, no,' I said, taken aback, 'You just saw him outside.'

'Actually, we didn't. We couldn't spot him. We didn't tell you because we didn't want to make you sad. He's not in here, is he?' She wondered in her well-thought-out way.

So, I answered as honestly as I could that Rudolph had a different job, which involved special, very special, deliveries, and would never become pie. The deer in the pie we were eating were specially farm-reared and treated well in the span of their lives. But we were meat-eaters, and as long as the process was humanely handled, legal and healthy, there was no difference between eating that and the ham they'd scoffed at breakfast or the chicken roasting for dinner that night.

They understood, for now at least, and that was enough. We wouldn't stand in the way of a change in lifestyle choice made when they were capable of informed and considered decisions. There was a delicious pie going cold, however, that would be an utter shame to waste. 'Well, if it isn't Rudolph ...' our son said to himself happily even as he pushed his spotless plate forward for seconds. No, not Rudolph, I thought, because he isn't real, but I didn't say. That would be for another day.

Of course we're as conflicted about these issues as the

next person. I have had a menagerie over the years but am unapologetically omnivorous. I started life with a kitten, then a much-loved dog, a friend's rooster that sadly died (we *really* had nothing to do with that and were in the most terrible quandary over how to prove it). Then, there was the sparrow with a broken wing, a baby bat that took to us, and so on. None of whom we ate but all of whom we might, if legally sourced and cooked right (okay, not the dog or cat). Yet, if the whole food chain conundrum confounds, then how much more confusing is everything connected with human life. And death. My son and I have discussed death in a context so close to home that it was pretty scary. For me.

'Mommy, you know I was awake through my operation and saw everything they were doing to me, don't you? It didn't frighten me though.' He confided one day, a few months after an operation to sort out water retention in an unfortunate place (but one that had excited him greatly at the beginning when he thought his equipment had grown to thrice its size overnight).

'Sweetheart,' I said to him the first time he mentioned it, 'I was there when they put you to sleep with a big whopping dose of general anaesthesia. You couldn't have been awake. You couldn't have seen anything.'

'I did though,' he said confidently. 'At first it went dark but when I woke, it was very bright and I felt floaty but could see everything. It was really interesting. Bet I could perform an operation now!' Yeah, that last bit – scary, huh? But he has stuck to his story, that he watched his own operation (and can provide details, though we'll never know how true). He has a fertile imagination, but wouldn't that need a prompt for something like this? And he has never, to my knowledge, come across the concept of out-of-body experiences. But come up with it he surely has. And gently laugh it off, we did.

Because family of heathens that we are, there is no such thing as an afterlife, except in the hearts of those we leave behind. And worryingly nowadays, in the digital world, where I still see friends who've died live on in comments and even glow green in the chat box. That last, I have once or twice used completely irrationally to reach out to them, knowing there would be no answer. Horrifyingly for someone I know, messaging a dead friend almost caused their own death from shock when said friend answered back. It turned out to be a very unfortunate prank, but it goes to show how death has become something we rub along with increasingly every day.

In 2012, over 30 million Facebook accounts belonged to the deceased, which suggests it will have become a digital graveyard with more of the departed than the living on its pages by 2065[70]. I don't need life after death because what I have now with my beautiful family and home, and the joy I derive from my work is heaven enough. Yet I'm also aware that it is all so fragile, it could shatter at any time. But disturbingly, as acutely aware of its constant presence is this generation of children.

'Dead people unsettle me,' said our little girl in her extremely grown-up way, 'because they are lost to us forever.'

'Yeah, *and* they turn into zombies,' offered her year-older brother.

'Very ill folks worry me too,' she continued thoughtfully, 'as they won't be around to make memories with much longer. That's terribly sad.'

'Yeah, AND they'll become zombies!' reminded our son.

Despite their very different takes on it, death is so much more a part of their lives than it was ours. The most popular children's book and film series of them all, *Harry Potter*, starts with death and ends with apocalyptic destruction, while video games normalize, even glorify such things. The most popular video games, played by 68 per cent of American households, don't deny having excessive 'blood and gore' in their contents. And though no conclusive link has been found between mass violence and video games, enough studies in recent years have established that players experience a short-term surge towards aggression after[71]. With guns, especially in the aforementioned country, being as easy to pick up as sweets were for us kids, is it any wonder there were sixty-four school shootings in 2015[72]? Or that kids around the world are more aware of the imminence of death than we ever were? But is the world a scarier place really?

Then	Now
Mass deaths: The Black Death, for example, wiped out 50 million in Europe while bringing out the very worst in mankind – irrational fear, strange superstitious practices, treachery and abominable cruelty to each other.	**Mass stupidity**: Wipes out innocent people around the world hourly. It could be gun crime in the US or femicide in India. It brings out the very worst in mankind: irrational fear of the 'other', strange superstitious practices, e.g., buying and believing in tabloid trash, talk of building nation-separating walls, treachery against one's own kind who support views contrary to your own, abominable cruelty to anyone 'different' in view or aspect.

Then	Now
The rack: Religious persecution by means most foul (e.g., this instrument) marked a particularly nasty period in history where people betrayed and murdered even their dearest in the name of religion. Greek or Roman in origin, it rose to fame in Medieval and Tudor England.	**Ba-rack**: He didn't start the religious wars raging around us today. But he hasn't been able to put out the fire previous US administrations have fanned with the help of greedy corporations, 'friendly' governments and religious extremists around the world. The body count is now, well, countless.
Civil war: Many, all over the world, throughout history. More damage to people, property and any chances of peace going forward than you can begin to tot up.	**Uncivil war**: Partly sprung from all that factional fighting of yore is today's dirty warfare. Drones, chemical bombs, civilian strikes, assassinations. Name anything terrible and underhand, and it now happens. Leaving vast numbers dead.
Buns: Marie Antoinette is supposed to have said, 'Let them eat cake!' when told of the famished state of the French whom she ruled with her husband Louis XVI. Mired in poverty, death, disease,	**Guns**: You really can't rant about guns enough, or the damage they do us daily. With little control over who has them (usually, and naturally, the bloodthirsty), gun crime is rife around the world. There were 353

Then	Now
discrimination and disenfranchisement while the royalty and nobility lived it up in obscene splendour, the French masses soon decided to take her advice and slice some ... no, not bread ... but head. Which is remembered as the French Revolution and its memorable mascot – La Guillotine.	mass shootings in the US in 2015. Yet, El Salvador, Honduras and Jamaica topped global firearm homicides lists[73] (imagine how commonplace there)! In India, we own 40 million guns, second only to the US (woohoo). Of those, 85 per cent are unregistered and involved in 90 per cent of gun murders.[74]
The rest. Oppression, famine, pestilence, superstition, quackery. And too little food.	**The rest.** Terrorism, paedophilia, drugs, serial killers, nukes, HIV. And too much food.
The verdict: Millions of deaths. Annually. With little action from the powers that be. Very grim.	**The verdict**: Millions of deaths. Annually. With little action from the powers that be. Very grim.

There are, it would appear, as many ways to die now as there were before. The world has always been hazardous, so why this heightened perception of death and danger currently? I blame the media and the social media. If it is a smaller world because of them, faraway terrors also feel closer to us than ever before. They do everything they can to frighten the bejesus out of us (because shaken, uncertain customers are returning customers, requiring reassurance and direction). So, now we're perpetually petrified. Of everything (Eeek! Ebola! Where, where? Right behind you, 5000 miles away).

None of these eventualities troubled the kids though. It wasn't even my father, their Dadu's imminent prostate operation that worried them. His operation worried me, but my kids were anxious about *my* health. Children have a sixth sense and can detect unrest. Mommy is worried. Mommy is not sleeping well. *And* Mommy had an epileptic fit one day! I've been doing it for so long, I'm very matter-of-fact about it. But it was a shock for the children. Oh, they knew I blacked out occasionally, but witnessing it frightened them. 'Mommy,' asked four-year-old Anika, her doe-eyes brimming, 'When you black out, do you die a little?'

It's been drilled into them through children's books and movies that losing a parent is a standard part of childhood. From Cinders and Mowgli to the sisters in Frozen, they have all lost parents before their stories even got started. And it can, kids are told, happen in the blink of an eye. Now you have mommy and now you don't! And so with my collapse, the idea of death as something close by had snuck up on them. Something that, ironically, lived and breathed, and lay in wait like the monsters under their beds. And this one with its curving scythe might be waiting for Mommy!

To grasp the extent of their anxiety, I tried to recall how I felt about death as a child. For the longest time, I didn't believe in it any more than I did fairies. It began with the death of my Dadadu or great-grandfather, a man I loved more than any other at that stage. He died in Kolkata while we lived in the Philippines. I was far enough away to get away with telling myself he hadn't died; he'd just taken his 'Shingara Gari' for a spin somewhere nice but distant. I taught myself to think of him with his walking stick and tweed suit, not wading through Kolkata floods to spend the afternoon with me, but off on an adventure on some enchanted highway. It was a pleasant thought and I was, after all, just eight. And like my confession about writing to dead digital friends, I continued to send letters to Kolkata to my favourite person in the world. Till we went home and I had to face the fact that he really wasn't there anymore.

In my mid-twenties, still a child in many ways, I moved to England and for nearly fifteen years after, thought of my parents as thirty-year-olds (even as I out-aged them). It's an easy cop-out when you're far from home and don't have to watch your loved ones age. So I froze them conveniently in time, forever thirty-odd, sitting around our dining table in the Philippines with a scrumptious spread before them, chatting about books and life. But, of course they are not, they are closer to seventy, and subject to the ravages of time. How much my father had aged struck me especially when neither his stomach nor his legs could keep up with the gastronomic exotica we consumed, or the hours we walked, on a trip to Paris. He may have carried on gamely but it was the start of the illnesses and operations that occasioned my worry and my children's cogitations on their own mother's death.

But death and disease don't always strike where expected. My children's ninety-eight-year-old paternal great-great-aunt, the apparently indestructible Aunty Nellie, was diagnosed with breast cancer soon after, shocking us all. After nearly a century of unfailingly good health, we had expected this strong, sturdy woman to walk off into the sunset unbowed and unaided. But the Big C struck like a bolt from the blue. And breast cancer does seem specially designed to cut tough, independent women down to size. Yet, not just breasts, almost every part of our vital, vivacious, life-giving bodies also deals us death.

Holes and bumps are what we women have, in which men want their stake (in every way). Additional holes and bumps are what we get when we fall ill, especially with 'women's illnesses'. Bumps are fibroids, polyps, stones and tumours, cancerous and otherwise. Holes are leaks, lesions, gashes, missing bits and more. Some life-threatening and some not. Like many other women, I've had my brushes with most of these. At sweet sixteen, I was given the gift of the knowledge that I had polycystic ovaries. Which explained the pain and discomfort I was going through, but as nothing could be done about them, I was told, they would neither improve nor allow me to have babies.

Eighteen years later, without any assistance (not counting 'squirms' from Hubby), I gave birth to first one and then two beautiful, bouncing babies. Last year, I finally had my perpetually painful, gallstone-packed (packed to bursting I tell you, there were hundreds of them) gall bladder removed, but only after five years of insisting I had them. And didn't want them. My doctor neither believed me nor wanted to have it checked. As women are twice as likely to develop gallstones as men because of the preponderance of oestrogen in their bodies, it's often dismissed as unimportant. Or even imaginary. Just like endometriosis, cholestasis, cervical cell anomalies, gestational diabetes, post-partum depression and perineal problems, which I've also had the good fortune to have. They are all 'women's problems', and all handled with similar degrees of indifference and disdain.

Women's lives have traditionally mattered less, so, women's health has been secondary. In India, men are not only more likely to be immunized in childhood than women, this gap has actually increased from 2.6 per cent to 3.8 per cent in recent years[75]. There is also a 37 per cent (and rising) disparity in healthcare expenditure on long-term illnesses in favour of men[76]. In Africa, women are more likely to contract AIDS because their sexual and reproductive health is neglected. Even in the US, more money is spent on men's than women's health (though the Republicans would contest this hotly). Of course, women are looked after as well as men in enlightened homes everywhere, but that, sadly, is just a small part of the world.

It doesn't help that quite often, women aren't taken very seriously when they are unwell. According to a new American Pain Report, 90 per cent of women who reported chronic pain felt their claims had been dismissed as illusory. Besides, it's a woman's lot to feel pain. Didn't Eve, that very real woman in that historically accurate book, bring it upon us? Shouldn't we just shut up and put up with it now, having so let mankind down? Why should science and medicine bother with our constant whinging anyway? Why should the world spend more money on the research and treatment of women's diseases, when we buy enough handbags already? And while these very valid questions are being asked, little is done to look into problems like endometriosis, which affects 176 million women worldwide, but isn't significant enough to have serious money invested in it.

Look at the cancers that women get: breast cancer is one of the biggest killers of women in the world. In 2012, another 1.7 million women were diagnosed with it. Half a million died from it in the same period. And today, a lot of money is invested in its detection and treatment, but only after women took the establishment – corporations, media and the medical fraternity, by the scruff of its neck in the eighties, and made it listen. Screenings became standard procedure in much of the western world as did fund-raising and mass awareness campaigns. As a result, breast cancer survival rates are increasing (having doubled in Britain since the seventies)[77].

But in the 'developing world', breast cancer *cases* have soared by 26 per cent in recent times. In India, 100,000 women are diagnosed with breast cancer annually, with a predicted rise to 131,000 by 2020[78]. With only 5 per cent of the global spending on cancer spread thinly over the larger but less prosperous parts of the world, the prognosis doesn't look good. In fact, worldwide investment in research on most of the diseases that women get more often than men – fibromyalgia, PCOS, dementia, arthritis, to name a few – is teeny-weeny (as teeny as the weenies of those who demur). So, why is that? It must be because we are making them up, right? It's our hysteria or perhaps nymphomania speaking. Maybe we just crave more attention from men. Instead of all this keeling over and dying from diseases we've concocted, we should get on with our most important job, which is to take care of men – pioneers, leaders and nation-builders that they are. That's all we've been asked to do, and we can't even get that right. Tsk.

Just like the early birds and bees talk the kids and I'd had, where a few things were delved into and others touched upon, to be taken up again when they're older, we discussed death. As a parent with two spooked sprogs, I had to find a silver lining for them. Put a happy spin on it so they wouldn't have nightmares. Especially with regard to their fears – unfounded – of the imminence of *my* death.

And there was, I found, something to cheer about. Mothers don't die that easy these days, I told them, explaining how advances in medical science had made it possible for people to live longer lives. In the last century, in the prosperous places of the world, life expectancy had increased by almost forty years. As recently as 1980, if you lived till seventy-nine, you would have lived to a grand old age. By 2010, it was almost the norm to live to your eighties. And in 2050? They predict 4.1 million centenarians that year.

The irony is that even as we become aware of death earlier than ever, death itself has been postponed for most. A long life spent mulling over mortality is not an attractive prospect, but I kept that thought to myself. Instead, I talked frankly about my fainting fits. When I swoon, I told my kids, I have lit-up dreams, like Joan of Arc's visions from God. Mine are certainly not from God, it's just my brain taking an enforced break. I am not dying. Not even a little. Recent research does suggest those afflicted with epilepsy are eleven times more likely to die prematurely. They are also three times more likely to commit suicide. And if that wasn't enough, half of all epileptic deaths happened to the under-fifty-fives. None of which I told the kids.

What I did say was: Look, Mommy hardly ever has seizures. And seizures leading to falls and collisions are the main cause of deaths in epileptics. Mommy more often swoons (rather prettily if I say so myself) than spasms, and that isn't half as dangerous!

Finally, to make them feel less helpless, I taught them how best to deal with situations that struck them as scary – me blacking out, one of them having an accident, their father being bested in his annual fight with the Christmas tree. That sort of thing. I talked them through making emergency calls to save the day in those circumstances. They were excited at the idea of being 'superheroes'. 'Rohan Stormchild and Anika Lightningquick,' I said to them, 'I have every intention of living till a 105. Bet you won't like it when Mommy's still trying to cuddle you when you're seventy-one!'

'Ewww', they'd ordinarily say to something like that, 'we'd

be far too old for cuddles!' This time though, they drew me into a scrum. Then my little girl whispered in my ear, 'We're never gonna let go, Mommy. We shall buy the house next door and dig a tunnel underneath so we can get to you super-quick when you need us.' Oh dear, I thought to myself, will I never have peace and quiet again, but also, what wonderful, beautiful little people you are and how proud I am of you!

As often as they turn the tables on Mommy by reassuring her when she thinks *they* are in need of comfort, there is one thing she can still do for them. When I tuck them in at night, I make a point of showing my disdain for the monsters under their beds. I show my children that Gruff, Huff, Gribbles, and even that new one with the scythe, don't bother me and shouldn't worry them. Mommy can totally take on their monsters, even if she can't always slay her own.

16

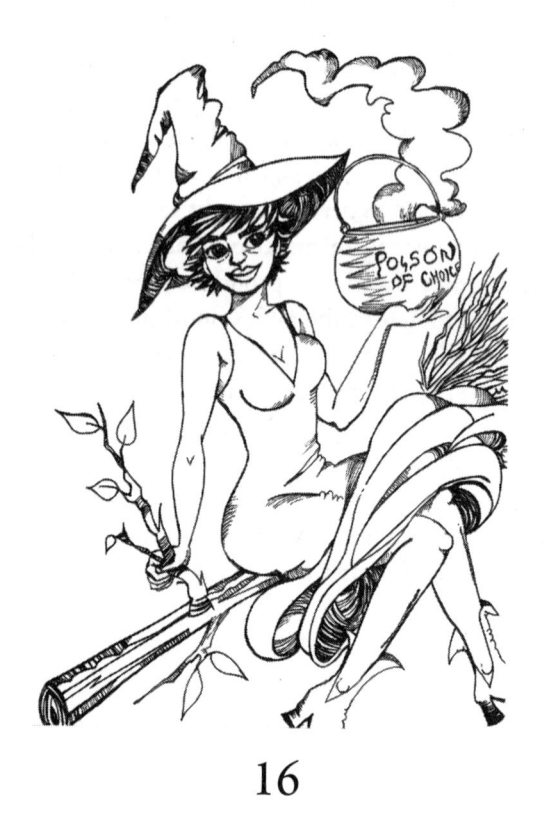

Meltdowns for Mommies

Sherwood Forest was still. With spring in the air, there was no crunch of footsteps on frosty ground or the wind shrieking through the trees. That late afternoon was silent, with even the scratch-scratch-scratch of squirrels hunting for nuts done for the day, and the birds flown as the smell of dusk rolled in. The luminescent green of tree and shrubbery, gilded by the sun at its zenith, was turning a more thoughtful shade. A quieter hue.

Quiet would not be the term I'd use for my life. Hue, as in hue and cry as well as colour, would be a better word to associate with it. Neither all good nor bad but with plenty of drama – eventful is what I'd call it. And I'm fast coming to the conclusion that this is how life will be, because this is who I am. Too unsettled to be contented but also, too aware of the hilarity of it all to play the tragic heroine. Not a 'happening' person, mind (maybe that, hopefully that, when I've got a few books out), but an 'eventful' person, someone stuff (shitloads of it) happens to. And that is bound to continue. What gives me this uncanny hunch you ask?

Well, how about the last few years, leading up to and into my forties, as a harbinger of things to come. As you've seen, what could have been a quiet entrance into a new decade became this huge production: death, heartbreak, and curl-up-in-a-corner despair, but also overwhelming joy, all-conquering love and moments of pure, crystalline perfection. Moments like those spent with my family in our garden at summertime, quiet and unexceptional to those who may take for granted the things I couldn't after the journey I'd had, but flawless to me.

With the kids rolling down small swells, climbing walnut trees and sneaking up on the irritable, iridescent pheasants that flock to our garden on sunny days, their father and I might shake our heads at their boisterous antics and exchange a rueful smile. Sometimes those rueful smiles would deepen into looks of profound love, exchanged fleetingly as he fired up the wood stove and I clumsily skewered the chicken, diced mango and red pepper. But the feeling was far from fleeting, and stayed even when our eyes unlocked and slid back to the tasks at hand, sometimes called 'kids'.

On the other end of the spectrum from these moments of quiet satisfaction was the song and dance of my arrival at my fourth decade, with encores too of every mistake along the way. What's that condition called when we obdurately hold out against learning from life? Oh yeah, stupidity. Stupid is not the impression most people have of me and I'm not here to convince you otherwise, but post-miscarriage, post-postpartum depression, neither of which I could have helped, I wallowed in sorrow, I reached out to the wrong people (misjudging men had always been my special talent), I lost any deference for discretion I may have had and launched into a more extravagant public meltdown than even Britney managed. All of which I could have averted.

Alongside the deep despair and feelings of emptiness I became prey to after my miscarriage in the run-up to my fortieth year, other unhappy symptoms sprang up. Under pressure, I would sometimes feel claustrophobic to the extent that the walls would appear to close in on me, the breath would be squeezed from my body and I would, panic-stricken, look around for an exit. Not just from the steadily shrinking room, which I knew was an illusion, but out of my own skin. This panic, combined with a sore-picking dwelling on unhappy, unknowable things, and the resulting need to cry bitterly and throw myself about (the last of which I never did, deciding it was way too Mrs Rochester), were classic anxiety-attack symptoms which I displayed in spades, but did not know anything about or how to manage till months later.

When I discovered what it might be, I drew on experience and received wisdom to help me cope, rather than hauling my crazy (but once again firm) ass to a psychiatrist as I should have. My family's long-standing association with them had made me averse to their seemingly hit-and-miss treatments (the *New England Journal of Medicine* in 2008 found that antidepressants only worked half the time). But my Bearded Boy's death sent me spiralling into depths of depression I wasn't sure I could emerge from on my own. So I finally relented, darkening a head doctor's door soon after.

'Do you sleep a lot? Sure sign of depression,' he nodded wisely.

'No, I don't sleep much at all, there's always so much going on in my head ...'

'Sure sign of depression.' He repeated, nodding, and prescribed a raft of pills.

Because it was a raft, a life-saving device in the bottomless sea I was drowning in, I started taking them. That's when I hit rock-bottom. The panic attacks worsened. On one occasion, I had to crawl out of the door to fetch my children from school at home-time because there was something solid, like a brick wall that moved where I did, blocking my way. I crawled because the wall was stupid; it hadn't thought to extend itself to the floor. Once I'd got past the front door, breathed in fresh air and calm, I proceeded to the school as a biped normally would, and no one was the wiser. I knew though. I knew how low I'd sunk (literally) and the pills were given the heave-ho soon after (don't try this at home, kids, it may not be right for you).

I have never crawled out the front door since. Or cried as bitterly. Or worried about turning into Mrs Rochester ever again. I was suddenly much happier, more in control and raring to get on with things. Of course, it had nothing to do with the pills I'd taken briefly before giving them up. Given up because the time felt right. The post-partum fog that had clung to me for nearly three years was lifting. Or that *something else* that had been brewing through it all was bubbling to the top.

The year of my miscarriage had seen other upheavals. The husband's new job, first-time nursery for the kids, and something new was happening to me too. An unstoppable tide of feelings that assailed me and then came tumbling out. I wanted to reach out to people, to make them understand who I was, what I felt ... the agony I was in. For that I needed to write. Constantly. Serendipitously at just that time, along came the best-known British broadsheet asking me to write about Indian womanhood. I know that one well, I thought happily (as happily as one can in the throes of depression).

Out cascaded every splendid thing that had ever happened to me. And each horrible one too. Up they came like vomit. I wrote about vomiting in church as a child and the chastisement that followed. About swooning my way through my growing years. And finally, about the abuse I'd endured in my first marriage, which very few knew about. Then *everybody* did. Because I was writing for nearly everyone by then – English papers, Indian magazines and Australian websites. They all seemed to want, unexpectedly, gratifyingly, a piece of my funny-sad-weird confessional pie. I was soon being urged to put it together in a book (and voilà). But as the interest trebled, so did the mess.

The down side of this shouting from the rooftops about bodily phenomena – parts, fluids and flings, was that people jumped to unfortunate conclusions about me. In Kolkata after the Philippines, and then again in Delhi, the whisper that had followed me around was the 'what kind of a girl is she' hiss, said with rolling eyes and indrawn breath to express the full extent of their horror at my ways. Well, I got more of that when I opened up to the world fifteen years later. 'Damaged goods' and 'hysterical' (maybe they meant ha-ha?) were things I heard but also heart-warmingly, 'brave', 'tenacious' and even the humbling 'inspirational' from women who felt encouraged by my admissions to come out with their own. It was the kind of validation I desperately needed at that fragile stage of life. I felt nothing good about myself despite the triumphs I was totting up, so I needed others to feel good for me instead. But in with the support, came a torrent of sleaze.

Laughing with a virtual man who seemed intelligent and urbane, 'Oh, I have very firm opinions!' I said. 'What else about you is firm?' he slimed in return, 'Your pictures tell me your breasts must be.'

And from another fella: 'I had a dream about you last night. You were in white socks and nothing else,' he perved, 'on your hands and knees in my bedroom wardrobe where I found you. And fucked you.'

Needless to say, some of these 'friends' were summarily despatched. But others I kept on because a lot of the time they said the right things. Stuff that helped me get through the day when the family was away and I was left with my morbid thoughts (and mountains of housework, but when has that ever engaged the mind?). Amongst them was one man, a man who not only said all the right things, but seemed to genuinely care.

Sweeping into my life in an unthreatening avuncular manner, this close friend of a trusted family friend shook out his big, fluffy angelic wings and tucked me under them with a paternal love that was not only unexpected and deeply warming, but also just what I needed at that stage in my life. This was a depression-fuelled phase of my life where I felt I required hourly validation and affection, which neither my newly school-going children nor my loving but hard-working (therefore not available to me in the course of the day) husband could give me. But this man appeared to be offering me exactly that.

Soon, I had let my guard down and was luxuriating in

this 'other' love. As he got closer and closer and words of love began to be said, I told him what I had been through in the past. And how fragile I still was as a result. I shared how important it was to me that any close association be founded on a framework of respect for, and acceptance of, my need for honesty, transparency and integrity. He promised it would be so. And I let him into my life on that basis. Very quickly he became part of the family, though remotely. My husband knew all about him. And The Man listened with what seemed like fond interest to stories of the children. He loved everything I wrote. He waxed lyrical over the beauty of my eyes. He praised me to the skies for the courage with which I carried on in the face of adversity – my depression, the epilepsy, isolation in beautiful Sherwood Forest (a boon that felt less like one at the time), and inability to cook shellfish. Nobody gets me like this man I thought, and I allowed him in as close as close can be in a virtual relationship.

But you know where I am going with this story, don't you? Of course none of it was real. Neither the love nor the understanding or the 'honesty'. The end came very suddenly too. The day after I went under the knife for another of my lingering post-natal problems, he decided to end the association with a great deal of nastiness followed by a chilling silence. An unexpected development considering I had, just the week before, attempted to finish with him on the grounds that it no longer felt right. It had been on the turn for a few weeks, from a warm and comforting connection to a sordid game of smoke and mirrors. He persuaded me that wasn't so, and that it would all work out. That he wasn't 'ready'.

After his vanishing act, I found out what it was he had suddenly become 'ready' for, as other women he had comforted through crises, professed vast amounts of admiration for, and promised undying *exclusive* love to (to all, simultaneously), came tumbling out of dark corners and dingy closets to whisper their terrible secrets to me. But it was not that alone which messed me up at a time when I needed no further trauma. It was the feeling of invasive, gut-wrenching violation I took away from it all that made it worse.

Physical attentions forced upon you are not, after all, the only kind of defilement. An incursion into your emotional life without your informed consent, or with consent taken from you under false pretences, is violation too. And it took months to get over it, on top of everything else I was working my way through. But he himself had a mental illness as I found out. Did he not understand my situation despite our discussions about it? Or was he so engrossed in drawing succour for himself from wherever he could, that he had never really listened?

The vanishing act turned out to be temporary, but after a few more twists and turns this association was finally laid to rest in the unmarked grave it deserved. What remained was that in having been well and truly 'catfished', I learnt the hard way, that salvation would not come in the form of another person. Certainly not another brain-sick soul, because misery does *not* love mirror-image company. Medicine would not save me either (that's not to say it doesn't others or won't for me, if required again).

If I needed to hear how feisty I was, how funny a raconteur, how terrific a writer, to help me through the darkness, I would have to work towards it. And I had begun; with the loss of Baby, I had rediscovered my writing voice, ironically. I was now actively, sanely, working towards realizing all these things in which resided, I thought and not wrongly, my deliverance. No, scrap sanely, because I was pouring all my turmoil into my pieces. Even happy articles (which many were) pulsed with a nervous energy that might have made riveting reading, but also told me I hadn't healed. Not just from the lesions left by unfortunate online liaisons, but from all the turmoil of that summer.

When the initial tears of loss and then of anger and disgust at my own folly dried up, there were still tears over the tears I worried had affected my children. But this very public outpouring of grief, this mid-life-mommy meltdown in the media, saved me too. I arrived in the end, after Bearded Boy's death and many wrong turns, at a place where I was exorcising many of my demons through writing. My depression buddies, aka the catfish crew, those online chums I believed would help me feel better, had only depressed me further, and the pills hadn't worked because I didn't want them to. Oh, how complicated life was dithering into my forties.

In contrast, I had zoomed into my thirties with purpose. And the purpose was to be rid of my horrendous husband (yes, sigh, it is too often about men). But though I was bruised and bloodied, I was unbowed, less so than in the limp to my forties. Still married to George when I stepped into my thirties, I had much less that was good in my life but I had an abundance of hope. I shrugged things off easier, bounced back quicker, forgot faster, but that's the unthinking beauty of youth, I guess.

The dithering could also be down to the many horror stories and urban myths that have attached themselves to our fortieth milepost. The forties are seen as a watershed decade, a line in the sand of maturity that you cross once and for all, never to be tempted into juvenile tomfoolery again. Is it any wonder such dread and terror surrounds our passage into this unforgiving decade? And that so many messes are made for purely that reason – panic, because there's no turning back? Mine was due to a different concatenation of circumstances rather than the fear of impending maturity (because really, I had nothing to fear). But a mess, as you know, is what I made of it.

The rags are strewn with stories of spectacular celebrity meltdowns. More often than not on the road to, or in their forties, that rocky (as opposed to rock-n-roll-y) decade. It's not surprising as that's when they stop being seen as hot young things, becoming 'legends' (if they're lucky) or silver foxes (if they're men). But often, they're just shunted aside. And then the shit hits the fan. Except that it doesn't affect the fan at all, or the press, which revels in it. It tars the star instead.

Heidi Klum celebrated her fortieth with a string of infamous affairs, hangovers and bad hair days, which wrecked her marriage to singer Seal, and tarnished her alluringly aloof super-model image. Vanessa Paradis, poor thing, wasn't even allowed a meltdown of her own, because for her fortieth birthday, Johnny Depp presented her (and the world) with news of his affair with the barely legal Amber Heard (and we all know how that worked out). Demi Moore in her forties had a high profile break-up with Ashton Kutcher, leading to rehab, anorexia, scurrilous pap stories and the usual derision that accompanies a woman's failure to 'keep a man'. That trebled for her because she tried to snag one sixteen years younger.

Yet, for every Heidi or Demi, there are a hundred Tom Cruises, Boris Beckers and Charlie Sheens. Men get an itch at this age they must scratch, we're told. And they scratch on a seismic scale, fathering babies in broom cupboards, drinking tiger blood, courting arrest for beating up their old wives, beating down the door to court arresting new wives, championing kooky churches (psst, Scientology), not to mention the sheer volume of affairs, tantrums, benders and bad decisions.

But they're men, we're reminded. They can, because they're allowed to. We might roll our eyes, but we won't judge harshly. We may even smirk in part-admiration. Not so with women. Oh no. When a woman, especially a mature or 'matronly' one, puts a foot wrong, never mind going off the rails altogether, then all hell breaks loose. The tabloids get out their tar and brush, society spits feathers and even family and friends are reluctant to forgive.

What is it about women over forty that so gets the world's goat? And goat is exactly how older women are perceived. Knobbly kneed, bleary-eyed, bleating and bearded. But also, if you're well up on your Greek mythology, a symbol of lust. And isn't that what a quarter of the world (half of all men) feel for the attractive older woman: a mixture of revulsion, fascination, fear and lust? Think Mrs Robinson easing sheer stockings off her shapely legs as the gauche young graduate goggles at her from the doorway. Flaunting her still-enthralling sexuality when she should have retired in sackcloth and ashes to the shadows, she is the epitome of the older woman the world wants to do, and then condemn and degrade for having been done (or having done, if my sassy, sexy forty-plus female friends are anything to go by!).

Because she had the sensuality of a woman who had grown comfortable in her skin, and the smarts to use it to get what she wanted, Mrs Robinson had her comeuppance. Which is just how it should be, ask any khap panchayat! Older women are punished regularly by these kangaroo courts for sexual transgressions (i.e., deciding what to do with their own bodies). Had they been jaded old men, wouldn't there be applause instead of punishment for bedding a filly (a stable-full, if you please)? Society has actively promoted unions between older men and younger women, to the extent that a decade-older man is the norm in many countries (including the purportedly progressive US, UK and Australia, where it constitutes up to 12 per cent of marriages, compared to a miniscule 1 per cent the other way around).

My nearly-never-used seduction technique aside, Mrs Robinson and I have much in common. I am, after all, over forty now. And my husband is almost two years younger than me. A wholly unremarkable age gap had it been the other way around, it makes me a cougar and him a toy boy in the myopic eyes of the world. This is a fact that doesn't bother me in the least, and is the source of much hilarity in our home. It's true that Demi and Ashton's goings-on weren't the most dignified but Paul and Joanne Newman, with Paul the younger of the two, were the most perfect couple ever. As heartwarming as Sunil Dutt and Nargis. Then there's Hugh Jackman and his older wife to whom he's utterly devoted. And Tina Turner and her much-younger husband, who have had a long, successful run together after her hellish marriage to the older Ike.

The logic behind older men and younger women is simply that younger women breed better and older men can support that breeding financially. But how horribly atavistic. The world no longer works that way. Women can breed when they want (science can help when the body clock falters), if they want, and without handouts from men. Nor are younger men less sensitive, less supportive or less successful (earnings can fall after the age of fifty). There are as many good reasons to get behind older women (and get behind you can, we're so much more adventurous).

I'd rather be a cougar than a sugar daddy's darling. The su-dads I found (and maybe I found the wrong 'uns) were anything but sweet. Far from looking after me, as older men are supposed to with their young women, they spent their time knocking the stuffing or the confidence (or both) out of me. The younger men in my life, on the other hand, have gently and lovingly taken care of me (taken care, not taken charge). I'm happy for you if your sugar daddy is every bit as sugary and generous as Willy Wonka, and ... er ... as willilicious. But you keep 'em; I'll stick to my toy boys. Boy, I meant. Singular. Honest.

That 'older' women should be asexual is just the tip of the iceberg of all that's wrong with the world's views on forty-plus femmes. And where there's misrepresentation, there is mistreatment. Amongst the many misnomers pinned on us are 'hag', 'old bat', 'prune', 'old bag', and 'crone'. Then there's witch. I don't mind being called a witch. There are, after all, witches and then there are sexy, sassy, clever witches. But the latter is a very modern take on an ancient insult you would only hurl at a woman you wanted dead.

A few centuries ago, that epithet could have been used to fell any one of us quick-witted and comely forty-somethings. And not just us, but our baby sisters in their thirties too. Back then, we were all dispensable past the first flush of youth. And if we had minds we were prepared to speak, we were ripe for burning. My outspokenness would have surely singled me out for the stake!

We've all been brought up on testimonials to the wickedness of witches. Most fairy tales have the older, wiser (and frankly, sexier) woman as the regulatory witch, with a virginal younger woman as her witless victim and a man, any man (from woolly woodcutters to slightly suspect dwarves to blue-blooded necrophiliacs) as the ingénue's only hope. Young women are *not* witless (and rarely virginal these days, you schmucks) and older women, far from wicked. And the truth has begun to seep out. In Disney's *Maleficent*, we discover the much-maligned eponymous witch wasn't, in fact, the worst party pooper of all time; she was a wronged woman trying to get her own back on Sleeping Beauty's hitherto whiter-than-white scumbag dad.

In the real world, an estimated 9 million 'witches' were burnt, drowned, maimed and tortured for daring to flout convention in fourteenth to seventeenth century Europe. Seventeenth-century America picked up where Europe left off and the hysteria surrounding witches led to the stomach-turning Salem Witch Trials. What was the deal with witch-hunts, you may well ask. Their heinous crimes against society ranged from questioning patriarchal dictates, using their healing skills and their childlessness. Past childbearing age, they were able to wrest control of their bodies from their male-dominated communities. Not just their bodies, they regained control of their destinies too. They became healers, growers and dispensers of natural medicine, carers for their community. People went to them for help. They listened to what these women had to say. Soon, outraged (but also really frightened) men everywhere were scrambling to find a solution to this abomination. They decided to cast these women as sorceresses and their healing powers as Satanic. They then had them destroyed.

The combative older woman continues to be feared and mistreated around the world. So, in lady lovin' Saudi Arabia, witchery is still punishable by death. And in India, witch-hunts, often presided over by the khap panchayats, have claimed the lives of 2,500 generally older women between 1995 and 2009[79].

The wicked witches of the west are no longer for burning.

They are for side-lining. When sharp, charismatic, fifty-five-year-old BBC anchor Moira Stuart was forced to bow out, sixty-four-year-old John Humphrys of the TV quiz 'Mastermind' said, 'There do seem to be remarkably few women with a few lines on their faces presenting on television compared to the wrinkled men[80].' So Aunty, as the Beeb is affectionately known, doesn't, in fact, care for aunties. In films, doddering septuagenarian Harrison Ford continues to get macho main roles when still lissome, fifteen-years-younger Michelle Pfeiffer has been put out to pasture. In Bollywood, while most forty-something actresses are reduced to playing 'Maaaa' (often to forty-something men), fifty-year-old Salman Khan carries on with debutantes on screen (and off, I hear).

Yet who's really got the swag? A group of tough, glamorous, astute older actresses who are now clawing it back for us 'crones'. Relegated to character parts in the past, forty-plus powerhouses like Julia Roberts, Nicole Kidman and Salma Hayek not only get the best roles (making their own movies to ensure they do), but also out-sizzle their twenty-something counterparts on any given Sunday. And a decade ago, who would've thought actresses Helen Mirren and Isabella Rossellini could become the faces of cosmetic giants in their sixties?

In the real world of completely skewwhiff standards, ageing, balding, pot-bellied men trade in their much-hotter wives for flouncy young arm ornaments, even as their former partners are urged to give up on life and love, and retire to nunneries. Sorry, that was Henry VIII and his first queen, Katherine, in the sixteenth century. But hey, not much has changed. Powerful men like Donald Trump are still showing the way. Fat and full of himself like Ol' Henry, Trump has already side-lined two slightly older (though not older than him!) wives for younger ones, and can be guaranteed to do it again.

Women, witches, wicked, wotsitmatter; they all begin with 'w'. And wubbish. Okay, that doesn't start with 'w' but it means expendable. Like women past a certain age.

There is a strange dissonance about this. Patriarchal societies start denying a woman's sexuality and sex appeal just as she reaches her prime and blossoms into something better than fluffy, something close to magnificent. Women are said to hit their sexual peak in their mid to late thirties, when the business of child bearing is often done. Then they understand their bodies, know what they want done to them (less of the grabbing, for example), and after years of labouring under someone frequently chosen for them, want to pick their own lovers too.

And gosh, doesn't that freak us out? All that oomph bouncing off the walls, but none of it for the taking. Reserved for the man she desires, for a change. How very selfish. So they turn the tables on her by declaring her ugly, used-up, shrivelled. Her self-assured sexuality is lampooned as comically predatory. She is made the butt of jokes, a figure of ridicule. 'Mutton dressed as lamb' if she steps out in something other than a tent, flaunting her better-now-it's-fuller figure. 'Cougar' if she takes lovers when she should only have cake. And 'Mrs Robinson' if they happen to be younger (whattodo, only young men can keep up).

The truth is she is less mutton and more Mata Hari. All my mature female friends dazzle, where they once just twinkled. Even I, never pretty (but hey, always presentable), turn more heads than I did before. Coming home in a taxi after an evening with friends, my twenty-two-year-old cabbie of South Asian origin started flirting. To shut him up, I told him I had hit forty. He nearly crashed his car. 'Really?' he squeaked unhappily. 'But you are far too hot to be an auntyji'. Oh my poor boy, I almost said, forty-plus women are supposed to be attractive! It's a myth that we are gnarled and grouchy.

But our sizzle has little to do with looks. Because there's no doubt there's extra padding, silvery streaks and a grid's worth of lines where there wasn't before. My grid is on my midriff sloping off into the rainforests below, both of which have been hacked into far too often not to leave devastation behind. On the bright side, the extra padding in all the right places is a gift from Mother Nature (and Father Time, and I suppose I must thank *him* too) I don't intend to return. And on the inside (where we are told beauty resides but no one takes the trouble to look), what we have is the confidence that comes with knowing who we are and what we want from life. The determination to. Never. Be. Pushed. Around. Again. The bliss of glasses that are always half-full. Of our poison of choice and *not* what we've been told good girls oughta have. Oh, the joy of being a full-fledged, full-figured forty-plus woman at last!

'Would you like me to seduce you?' I turn to the toy boy. My husband. NOT the taxi driver. 'Yes Ma'am,' he grins and herds the kids in for a spot of telly. I sashay in after him, feeling rather sure of the sexy, sassy, clever witch that I am. When we're done, I stretch languorously, reaching out to touch him again with my fingertips. 'Not going anywhere,' he smiles, though half-asleep. I put on a robe and run down the stairs, checking on the children letting rip to 'Let it go' on the screen in the family room. Okay, only my daughter, but gloriously. My son has a faraway look on his face, which is not a bad thing; it means he's walking in the forests of his mind, twining together the next lines of another of his epic poems. They are fed, they are happily occupied, soon to be tucked into bed with their favourite books by their loving mom and dad.

I walk swiftly into the real forest that surrounds us. Sherwood of lore and legend. Sherwood of the rebellion I've always had in my blood and the passion I'm learning to focus on my beautiful family, and on them alone. Oh, and on our forest home too. Now glowing ruby-red in the light of the sinking sun, the trees whispering in the faintest breeze before they settle for the night. The birds have long gone and the bugs come out to play. Their distant chirrup makes me think of the weak whirr of my old laptop in my cosy, mishti-doi-coloured study. The study from which prodigious amounts of writing – my writing – has been emerging. And being read around the world. But most importantly, being read by you! This is more than I could have hoped for from life.

This is perfection.

Acknowledgements

This book, being a memoir, could obviously not have happened without the many characters that people it. But most of them were not involved with its writing, so I will name those who have been. First and foremost, I must thank my husband Stephen and our children for everything – the immense love, understanding and support. The cake and the hot chocolate too, to keep me going. My husband read the manuscript a number of times for me. But not the kids – not just yet! I would like to thank my parents Anindita and Prithwiraj, for all their love and encouragement, and for reading the manuscript and backing it, though it is not always complimentary about them! Of the friends who vetted sections and reassured me I was on the right track, I'd like to thank Suhrid Chattopadhyay, because it's not the first time he has provided a reading service and it won't be the last. Finally, to Arunava Sinha who first thought this could be a book, Karthika V.K. who commissioned it, and Ajitha G.S. who steered it to a safe port, I want to say – thank you!

References

1. Rachel Grate, 'Reign Proves There's No Masturbating On Network TV Allowed', https://mic.com/articles/69071/reign-proves-there-s-no-masturbating-on-network-tv-allowed#.j1TjUA2FW; Last accessed on 23 May 2017.
2. Therese Oneill, 'Masturbation Was Once Considered More Offensive Than Child Abuse', *The Week*, http://theweek.com/articles/453676/masturbation-once-considered-more-offensive-than-child-abuse; Last accessed on 23 May 2017.
3. Hugo Schwyzer, 'Vibrators and Clitoridectomies: How Victorian Doctors Took Control of Women's Orgasms', *Jezebel*, http://jezebel.com/5914350/vibrators-and-clitoridectomies-how-victorian-doctors-took-control-of-womens-orgasms; Last accessed on 2017.
4. Radhika Sanghani, 'Sexually Exploring Ourselves As Children Is Anything But Shameful, *Daily Life*, https://www.google.co.in/search?q=Sexually+exploring+ourselves+as+children+is+anything+but+shameful&oq=Sexually+exploring+ourselves+as+children+is+anything+but+ shameful&aqs=chrome..69i57.341i0i4&sourceid=chrome&ie=UTF-8; Last accessed on 23 May 2017.
5. 'Non-reproductive Sexual Behaviour in Animals', *Wikipedia*, https://en.wikipedia.org/wiki/Non-reproductive_sexual_behavior_in_animals; Last accessed on 23 May 2017.
6. Sigmund Freud, *Three Contributions to the Sexual Theory; The Infantile Sexuality 1910*.
7. Therese Oneill, 'Masturbation Was Once Considered More Offensive than Child Abuse', *The Week*, http://theweek.com/articles/453676/masturbation-once-considered-more-offensive-than-child-abuse; Last accessed on 24 May 2017.
8. Rupi Kaur, https://www.instagram.com/rupikaur_/?hl=en, Last accessed on 24 May 2017.

9. Sarah Barns and Bianca London, 'Women's Bodies Don't Exist for Public Consumption', *Mail Online*, http://www.dailymail.co.uk/femail/article-3201878/Runner-completed-London-Marathon-free-bleeding-hits-critics-uncomfortable-normal-process.html; Last accessed on 24 May 2107.
10. Hannah Betts, 'The P Word: A Last Taboo', *The Telegraph*, http://www.telegraph.co.uk/women/womens-life/10401952/Periods-A-last-taboo.-Why-the-hell-cant-we-talk-about-them.html; Last accessed on 27 May 2017.
11. Narayan Lakshman, 'UN Marks World Toilet Day' *The Hindu*, http://www.thehindu.com/sci-tech/health/policy-and-issues/un-marks-world-toilet-day/article5369040.ece; Last accessed on 24 May 2017.
12. Hannah Betts, 'The P Word: A Last Taboo', *The Telegraph*.
13. Vibeke Venema, 'The Indian Sanitary Pad Revolutionary', BBC World Service, http://www.bbc.com/news/magazine-26260978, Last accessed on 24 May 2017.
14. Shelly Walia, 'These Men are Fighting Menstruation Taboos in India – And Helping Women Leave Dirty Rags Behind', *Quartz India*, https://qz.com/412907/these-men-are-fighting-menstruation-taboos-in-india-and-helping-women-leave-dirty-rags-behind/; Last accessed on 24 May 2017.
15. David Smith, 'Jacob Zuma says it is not right for women to remain unmarried', *The Guardian*, https://www.theguardian.com/world/2012/aug/22/jacob-zuma-women-unmarried; Last accessed on 24 May 2017.
16. Deepshikha Ghosh, 'After Sakshi Maharaj, Bengal BJP Leader says "Hindus Should Have 5 Children"', NDTV.com, http://www.ndtv.com/india-news/after-sakshi-maharaj-bengal-bjp-leader-says-hindus-should-have-5-children-726826; Last accessed on 24 May 2017.
17. 'Blood Group Anomaly Could Explain Tudor King's Reproductive Problems and Tyrannical Behaviour', SMU Research News, http://blog.smu.edu/research/2011/03/07/

blood-group-anomaly-could-explain-tudor-kings-reproductive-problems-and-tyrannical-behavior/; Last accessed on 24 May 2017.
18. Electroconvulsive Therapy, Wikipedia, https://en.wikipedia.org/wiki/Electroconvulsive_therapy; Last accessed on 21 June 2017.
19. Helen Thomson, 'Study of Holocaust Survivors Finds Trauma Passed on to Children's Genes', *The Guardian*, https://www.theguardian.com/science/2015/aug/21/study-of-holocaust-survivors-finds-trauma-passed-on-to-childrens-genes; Last accessed on 21 June 2017.
20. 'Gender and Women's Mental Health' WHO, http://www.who.int/mental_health/prevention/genderwomen/en/; Last accessed on 21 June 2017.
21. 'Tina Fey Quotes', Goodreads, https://www.goodreads.com/author/quotes/4385839.Tina_Fey; Last accessed on 2017.
22. Dan Greenberg, '10 Mind-Boggling Psychiatric Treatments', *Mental Floss*, http://mentalfloss.com/article/31489/10-mind-boggling-psychiatric-treatments; Last accessed on 21 June 2017.
23. Maureen Dowd, 'Men Have Not Only Stopped Evolving – They're Devolving', *The Globe and Mail*, https://www.theglobeandmail.com/opinion/munk-debates/maureen-dowd-men-have-not-only-stopped-evolving-theyre-devolving/article15453662/; Last accessed on 21 June 2017.
24. Ricky Gervais, Twitter.
25. Kate Hodal, 'Thailand's Skin-whitening Craze Reaches Woman's Intimate Areas', *The Guardian*, https://www.theguardian.com/world/2012/sep/23/thailand-vaginal-whitening-wash; Last accessed on 21 June 2017.
26. Matt Ford, 'Racism and the Execution Chamber', *The Atlantic*, https://www.theatlantic.com/politics/archive/2014/06/race-and-the-death-penalty/373081/; Last accessed on 21 June 2017.
27. Geeta Pandey, '100 Women 2014', BBC News, http://www.

bbc.com/news/world-asia-india-29708612; Last accessed on 21 June 2017.
28. 'City Judge Calls Living-in Relationships an "Immoral" Western Export', *Mail Online India*, http://www.dailymail.co.uk/indiahome/indianews/article-2088043/City-judge-calls-living-relationships-immoral-Western-export.html; Last accessed on 21 June 2017.
29. 'Indian Judge Says Pre-marital Sex "Against Religion"', BBC News, http://www.bbc.com/news/world-asia-india-25618163; Last accessed on 21 June 2017.
30. Amit Anand Choudhary, 'Couple Living Together will be Presumed Married, Supreme Court Rules', *The Times of India*, http//www.google.co.in/search?q=Couple+living+together+will+be+presumed+married%2C+Supreme Court+rules&oq=Couple+living+together+will+be+presumed+married%2C+Supreme+Court+rules&aqs=chrome..69i57,420i0i4&sourceid=chrome&ie=UTF-8; Last accessed on 21 June 2017.
31. Shiva Devnath, 'Mumbai: Couples picked up from hotel rooms, charged with "public indecency"', *Mid-day*, http://www.mid-day.com/articles/mumbai-couples-picked-up-from-hotel-rooms-charged-with-public-indecency/16437186; Last accessed on 21 June 2017.
32. Jennifer Gotrik, 'India Domestic Abuse More Common in "Arranged" Marriages', *Women News Network*, https://womennewsnetwork.net/2011/09/12/india-domestic-abuse-arranged-marriages/; Last accessed on 21 June 2017.
33. 'AIIMS Doctor Commits Suicide, Blames "Gay" Husband, Also a Doctor', NDTV.com, https://www.google.co.in/search?q=AIIMS+Doctor+Commits+Suicide+%2C+Blames+%27Gay%27+Husband%2C+Also+a+Doctor&aqs=chrome..69i57.338i0i4&sourceid=chrome&ie=UTF-8; Last accessed on 21 June 2017.
34. Emma Batha, 'Special Report: The Punishment was Death by Stoning', *The Independent*, http://www.independent.co.uk/

news/world/politics/special-report-the-punishment-was-death-by-stoning-the-crime-having-a-mobile-phone-8846585.html; Last accessed on 21 June 2017.

35. 'Rape Victim Should Have Been Careful: Andhra Pradesh Congress Chief', *The Times of India*, http://timesofindia.indiatimes.com/india/Rape-victim-should-have-been-careful-Andhra-Pradesh-Congress-chief/articleshow/17748819.cms; Last accessed on 21 June 2017.

36. 'BJP Minister Ties Himself in Knots over Morality, *The Times of India*, http://epaper.timesofindia.com/Repository/getFiles.asp?Style=OliveXLib:LowLevelEntityToPrint_TOINEW&Type=text/html&Locale=english-skin-custom&Path=TOICH/2013/01/05&ID=Ar01301; Last accessed on 21 June 2017.

37. 'Women to Blame for Earthquakes, Says Iran Cleric', *The Guardian*, https://www.theguardian.com/world/2010/apr/19/women-blame-earthquakes-iran-cleric; Last accessed on 21 June 2017.

38. Pat Robertson in Wikiquote.

39. '8 Quotes That Prove Jennifer Lopez Is the Queen Of Body Confidence', *Marie Claire*, http://www.marieclaire.co.uk/news/beauty-news/jennifer-lopez-body-quotes-118759; Last accessed on 21 June 2017.

40. *Hollywood Honey* in Cosmopolitan.

41. 'Obama Apology: US Media React to Kamala Harris "Sexism" Row', BBC News, http://www.bbc.com/news/world-us-canada-22050548; Last accessed on 21 June 2017.

42. 'Shame and Survival by Monica Lewinsky', *Vanity Fair*, http://www.vanityfair.com/style/society/2014/06/monica-lewinsky-humiliation-culture; Last accessed on 21 June 2017.

43. Lisa Clarke, 'Mostly Harmless? I Beg to Differ', *The Huffington Post*, http://www.huffingtonpost.co.uk/lisa-clarke/page-three-mostly-harmless-i-beg-to-differ_b_3034030.html; Last accessed on 21 June 2017.

44. 'Doctors Say Looking at Busty Women for 10 Minutes a Day Is Good for Your Health' *Daily Record*, http://www.dailyrecord.co.uk/news/health/doctors-say-looking-busty-women-1107578; Last accessed on 21 June 2017.
45. Sam Marsden, 'Angelina Jolie: I Had a Double Mastectomy to Reduce My Breast Cancer Risk', *The Telegraph UK*, https://www.google.co.in/search?q=Angelina+Jolie%3A+I+had+a+double+mastectomy+to+reduce+my+breast+cancer+risk&oq=Angelina+Jolie%3A+I+had+a+double+mastectomy+to+reduce+my+breast+ cancer+risk&aqs=chrome..69i57.216i0i 4&sourceid=chrome&ie=UTF-8; Last accessed on 21 June 2017.
46. Wendy Watson, 'Why Angelina Will Never Regret Sacrificing Her Breasts – by the First Woman in Britain to Do It', *Mail Online*, http://www.dailymail.co.uk/femail/article-2325203/Why-Angelina-Jolie-regret-sacrificing-breasts-woman-Britain-it.html; Last accessed on 21 June 2017.
47. 'What Are Eating Disorders?', NEDA, https://www.nationaleatingdisorders.org/learn/general-information/what-are-eating-disorders; Last accessed on 21 June 2017.
48. 'What is Obstetric Cholestasis?', British Liver Trust, https://www.britishlivertrust.org.uk/liver-information/liver-conditions/obstetric-cholestasis/; Last accessed on 21 June 2017.
49. Jennifer Thomson, 'A Court Just Made a Landmark Ruling for Abortion Rights in Northern Ireland', *The Conversation*, https//www.google.co.in/search?q=A+court+just+made+a+landmark+ruling+for+abortion+rights+in+Northern+Ireland+by+Jennifer+Thomson+The+Conversation&oq=A+court+just+made+a+landmark+ruling+for+abortion+rights+in+Northern+Ireland+by+Jennifer+Thomson+in+The+Converation&aqs=chrome..69i57i69i 6413.300i0i4&sourceid=chrome&ie=UTF-8; Last accessed on 21 June 2017.
50. 'Anti-abortion Violence' Wikipedia.

51. Tracie Egan Morrissey, 'Real Housewife Melissa Gorga's New Book Advocates Marital Rape', *Jezebel*, http://jezebel.com/real-housewife-melissa-gorgas-new-book-advocates-mar-1371722729; Last accessed on 21 June 2017.
52. Libby Brooks, 'The Campaign for Real Sex', *The Guardian*, https://www.theguardian.com/commentisfree/2006/jun/27/thecampaignforrealsex; Last accessed on 21 June 2017.
53. Alex Fletcher, 'Real Sex Season: Channel 4 Examines Pornography with New Shows', *Digital Spy*, http://www.digitalspy.com/tv/news/a506634/real-sex-season-channel-4-examines-pornography-with-new-shows/; Last accessed on 21 June 2017.
54. Mohd Faisal Fareed, 'Mulayam's shocker: Boys will be boys', *Indian Express*, http://indianexpress.com/article/india/politics/mulayam-singh-yadav-questions-death-penalty-for-rape-says-boys-make-mistakes/; Last accessed on 21 June 2017.
55. Matt Pearce, '"Boys will be boys" No Excuse; feds Target Montana Handling of Rapes', *Los Angeles Times*, http://www.latimes.com/nation/nationnow/la-na-nn-montana-rape-case-sexism-justice-20140217-story.html; Last accessed on 21 June 2017.
56. 'Russian Gay Propaganda Law', Wikipedia.
57. 'FAQ: What is Section 377?', Rediff News.
58. 'How Many More Will Die For Saying "I Love You"?' by Guest Writer in Human Rights Now Blog on Amnesty International, http://blog.amnestyusa.org/africa/how-many-more-will-die-for-saying-i-love-you/; Last accessed on 21 June 2017.
59. 'Homosexual Behaviour in Animals', Wikipedia.
60. 'Zac Efron on "Awkward" Dating', RTE.
61. Olivia Blair, 'Why are Some Women Never Able to Orgasm?', the *Independent*, http://www.independent.co.uk/life-style/love-sex/female-orgasm-women-disorder-why-cant-i-male-intercourse-explained-a7562296.html; Last accessed on 21 June 2017.

62. Jonathan Duffy, 'Britain's Secret Sex Survey', *BBC News*, https://www.google.co.in/search?q=Britain%27s+secret+sex+survey+by+Jonathan+Duffy+on+BBC+News&oq=Britain%27s+secret+sex+survey+by+Jonathan+Duffy+on+BBC+News&aqs=chrome..69i57.334 i0i 4&sourceid=chrome&ie=UTF-8; Last accessed on 21 June 2017.
63. Michael Castleman, 'The Most Important Sexual Statistic', *Psychology Today*, https://www.psychologytoday.com/blog/all-about-sex/200903/the-most-important-sexual-statistic; Last accessed on 21 June 2017.
64. Rachel Moss, '7 Famous Women Get Real About Female Masturbation', *Huffington Post*, http://www.huffingtonpost.co.uk/entry/celebrities-open-up-about-female-masturbation_uk_57dbce03e4b028e52a105008; Last accessed on 21 June 2017.
65. 'Breastfeeding', UNICEF, https://www.unicef.org/nutrition/index_24824.html; Last accessed on 21 June 2017.
66. 'Toplessness', Wikipedia.
67. Alexis Evans, 'Women Bare Their Naked Rumps to Protest Donald Trump', *Law Street Media*, https://lawstreetmedia.com/elections/women-bare-rumps-protest-trump/; Last accessed on 21 June 2017.
68. Nigel Wallace, 'Hundreds Strip Off on Brighton Beach for Topless "Free the Nipple" Protest', *the Mirror*, http://www.mirror.co.uk/news/weird-news/hundreds-strip-brighton-beach-topless-8146392; Last accessed on 21 June 2017.
69. Tridip K. Mandal, 'On Mother's Day, We Salute the Naked Protest of Manipur's Mothers', *The Quint*, https://www.google.co.in/search?q=On+Mother%E2%80%99s+Day%2+We+Salute+the+Naked+Protest+of+Manipur%E2%80%99s+Mothers+by+Tridip+K+Mandal+in+The+Quint&oq=On+Mother%E2%80%99s+Day%2C+We+Salute+theWe+Salute+the+Naked+

Protest+of+Manipur%E2%80%99s+Mothers+by+Tridip+K+Mandal+in+The+Quint&aqs=chrome..69i57.289i0i4&sourceid=chrome&ie=UTF-8; Last accessed on 21 June 2017.

70. Michael Hiscock, 'Dead Facebook Users will Soon Outnumber the Living', *The Loop*, http://www.theloop.ca/dead-facebook-users-will-soon-outnumber-the-living/; Last accessed on 21 June 2017.

71. Pete Etchells, 'What Is the Link Between Violent Video Games and Aggression?', *The Guardian*, https://www.theguardian.com/science/head-quarters/2013/sep/19/neuroscience-psychology; Last accessed on 21 June 2017.

72. 'Guns in the US: The Statistics Behind the Violence', *BBC News*, http://www.bbc.com/news/world-us-canada-34996604; Last accessed on 21 June 2017.

73. Mona Chalabi, 'Gun Homicides and Gun Ownership Listed by Country', *The Guardian*, https://www.theguardian.com/news/datablog/2012/jul/22/gun-homicides-ownership-world-list; Last accessed on 21 June 2017.

74. Mark Magnier, 'Gun Culture Spreads in India' *Los Angeles Times*, http://articles.latimes.com/2012/feb/20/world/la-fg-india-guns-20120221; Last accessed on 21 June 2017.

75. Yarlini Balarajan, S. Selvaraj and S.V. Subramanian, 'Health care and equity in India', www.ncbi.nlm.nih.gov, https://www.ncbi.nlm.nih.gov/pmc/articles/PMC3093249/; Last accessed on 21 June 2017.

76. G.S. Mudur, 'Even Educated Spend Less on Women Health – Scientists Surprised at Increasing Gender Gap in Expenditure on Illnesses', *The Telegraph India*, https://www.telegraphindia.com/1160718/jsp/nation/story_97320.jsp; Last accessed on 2017. Last accessed on 21 June 2017.

77. 'Breast Cancer Statistics' on World Cancer Research Fund International and Cancer Research, UK.

78. Arafat Tfayli, Sally Temraz, Rachel Abou Mrad and Ali

Shamseddine, 'Breast Cancer in Low- and Middle-Income Countries: An Emerging and Challenging Epidemic', on www.ncbi.nlm.nih.gov, https://www.ncbi.nlm.nih.gov/pmc/articles/PMC3010663/; Last accessed on 21 June 2017.
79. 'Witch-hunt', Wikipedia.
80. Richard Alleyne, 'BBC Accused of Ageism and Sexism after Stuart is Axed', *The Telegraph*, https://www.google.co.in/ search?q=BBC+accused+of+ageism+and+sexism+after+Stuart+is+axed+by+Richard+Alleyne+in+The+Telegraph&oq=BBC+accsed+of+ageism+and+sexism+after+Stuart+is+axed+by+Richard+Alleyne+in+The+Telegraph&aqs=chrome..69i57.287i0i4&sourceid=chrome&ie=UTF-8; Last accessed on 21 June 2017.

Besides the references listed above, the statistics used in this book are from commonly used online sources, in many cases appearing on multiple platforms. Like the book itself, there is no attempt to present them as scholarly, or as absolutes. They are useful indicators of global trends.

I have also drawn sections from my own published writing for *CNN-IBN*, *Times of India* and the *National Geographic Traveller India*.